ESSENTIAL OILS AND AROMATHERAPY:

AN INTRODUCTORY GUIDE

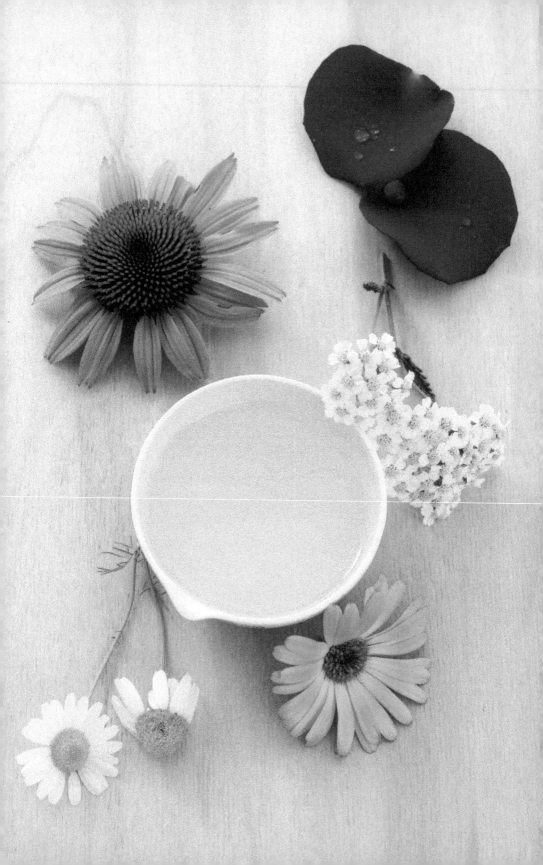

Essential Oils and Aromatherapy

An Introductory Guide

MORE THAN 300 RECIPES FOR HEALTH,
HOME, AND BEAUTY

SONOMA
PRESS

Photo credits: Masterfile, p.ii; Alena Haurylik/Shutterstock, p.vi; Hitdelight/Shutterstock, p.3; [no name]/Masterfile, p.4; photo division/Media Bakery, p.6; mountainpix/Shutterstock, p.11; Image Point Fr/Shutterstock, p.14; Lidante/Shutterstock, p.17; sai0112/Shutterstock, p.18; Anna Nemoy/Stocksy, p.27; Gts/Shutterstock, p.30 (left); Dream79/Shutterstock, p.30 (center); Petr Baumann/Shutterstock, p.30 (right); Serena Carminati/Shutterstock, p.35; Bernard Radvaner/Media Bakery, p.38; auremar/Shutterstock, p.47; Apollofoto/Shutterstock, p.48; stockcam/iStockphoto, p.51; Debu55y/Shutterstock, p.52; Melpomene/Shutterstock, p.54; Rhonda Adkins/Stocksy, p.57; ballycroy/iStockphoto, p.63; DUSAN ZIDAR/Shutterstock, p.70; hsvrs/iStockphoto, p.77; shmel/iStockphoto, p.83; CGissemann/iStockphoto, p.91; zkruger/Shutterstock, p.96; mama_mia/Shutterstock, p.105; bhofack2/iStockphoto, p.112; Elenathewise/iStockphoto, p.121; Irina Shomova/Shutterstock, p.128; Kirsty Begg/Stocksy, p.137; lynea/Shutterstock, p.144; grafvision/Shutterstock, p.151; Liv friis-larsen/Shutterstock, p.156; jirkaejc/Veer, p.163; Sea Wave/Shutterstock, p.177; matka_Wariatka/Shutterstock, p.182; amphotora/iStockphoto, p.191; joannawnuk/Shutterstock, p.199; Anna Ewa Bieniek/Shutterstock, p.202; zoryanchik/Shutterstock, p.208; matka_Wariatka/Shutterstock, p.214; JPC-PROD/Shutterstock, p.220; Masterfile, p.229; Natalia Klenova/Shutterstock, p.235; HandmadePictures/Shutterstock, p.240; Gita Kulinitch Studio/Shutterstock, p.247; barol16/iStockphoto, p.252; Serena Carminati/Shutterstock, p.261; unpict/Shutterstock, p.266; Ulrike Koeb/Stockfood, p.275; Christian Jung/Shutterstock, p.282; marylooo/Shutterstock, p.291; Elena Ray/Shutterstock, p.298; LazingBee/iStockphoto, p.305; Hitdelight/Shutterstock, p.310

ISBN: Print 978-0-98955-869-3

CONTENTS

1   Introduction

PART 1

5   Understanding Essential Oils

6   Chapter One: Learn the Basics

18   Chapter Two: Tools for Safe Healing

38   Chapter Three: Master the Methods

PART 2

53   Nature's Prescriptions

54   Chapter Four: A World of Natural Wellness

198 Chapter Five: Wellness and Beauty Boosts

214 Chapter Six: Simple Scents and Pleasures

220 Chapter Seven: Your Natural Home

228 Chapter Eight: Your Personal Apothecary

311 Appendix A: Top 25 Essential Oils and How to Use Them

314 Appendix B: Know Your Brands

317 Glossary

320 Additional Reading

326 Essential Oils and Carrier Oils Index

331 Remedies and Recipes Index

335 Index

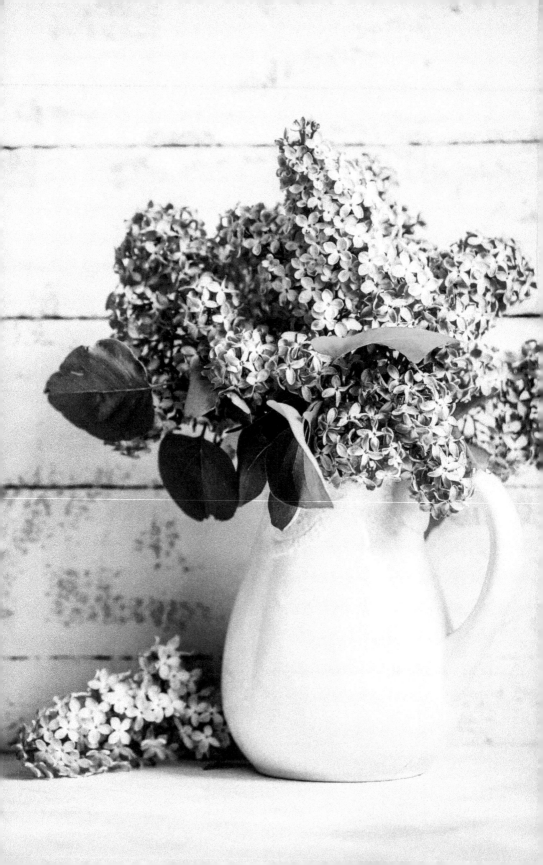

INTRODUCTION

Have you ever walked into a park in late spring and caught the scent of the first blooming lilacs or honeysuckle? Different regions have different plants, but people's reactions are almost universal: the sudden thrill at a familiar perfume, an immediate uplift in mood, an automatic smile, and often a sigh of relaxation. Maybe the fragrance of a flower in bloom announces that spring has arrived or brings back memories of a favorite garden, or maybe the scent has a healing power of its own. But the feeling of being happier and more relaxed is the same, no matter how it's explained. That walk in the park amounts to a brief experience of aromatherapy, one of the many uses to which essential oils have been put for almost a thousand years.

Today essential oils are largely relegated to a subordinate place in the Western apothecary, but they're still prevalent in the Ayurvedic medical practices of India and other Eastern cultures, and essential oils are also regulated and used as prescription medicines in several European countries, with results that have brought about something of a 21st-century revival for many of these scented wonders as some academic researchers begin to test their effects. And with health care costs skyrocketing, it's no surprise that many people are exploring ways to remedy some of their own common ailments without running to the doctor over and over and racking up medical bills for minor problems. Natural disasters seem to be coming more frequently, too, which is why people everywhere are starting to see essential oils as an important component of a preparedness kit for times when there's no access to prescription medications.

But it's important to know which essential oils are helpful for which conditions, and it's just as important to know exactly how essential oils should be used. This book explains what essential oils are and teaches you how to use them in aromatherapy and in topical applications for more than 100 ailments. It also includes recipes for making your own massage oils and cosmetics as well as sachets, scented bath products, candles, and nontoxic household cleaners. And Appendix A lists the 25 most common essential oils along with the conditions each oil treats.

If you have a major illness, there's no substitute for modern medicine. But essential oils can give you the power to take control of your daily health and manage many common ailments. This book puts the tools and techniques right in your hands.

BEFORE YOU BEGIN

Once you start exploring, you'll find a lot of information about essential oils online. You'll find a lot of misinformation, too, such as the notion that the term *therapeutic-grade essential oil* is anything more than a branding slogan invented by multi-level marketers of these products, or the legend that medieval Europeans warded off bubonic plague by wearing masks filled with "antiviral" aromatic herbs (the herbs probably did help with the stench of plague-stricken cities and towns).

Sooner or later you'll also see reports that people in some countries take essential oils internally—a piece of information that happens to be true, especially in France, where essential oils are sometimes prescribed for oral use, but only under strict medical supervision, and with prescriptions filled by pharmacists specially trained in the oils' properties, interactions, and side effects.

In the United States, though, no regulatory body inspects or controls the essential oils sold in stores or through distributors, and there are no established standards for a therapeutic dose. **This book strongly advises you not to take any essential oil internally**—not to place any oil in your mouth or under your tongue, not to swallow any oil or put it in your eyes or your ears, and not to use a syringe to inject any oil into your body or any body cavity through any opening.

Why take a chance with your health? Talk with your doctor before using any essential oil. And if your doctor tells you it's not safe to use essential oils internally, you can still enjoy their benefits through inhalation and topical application.

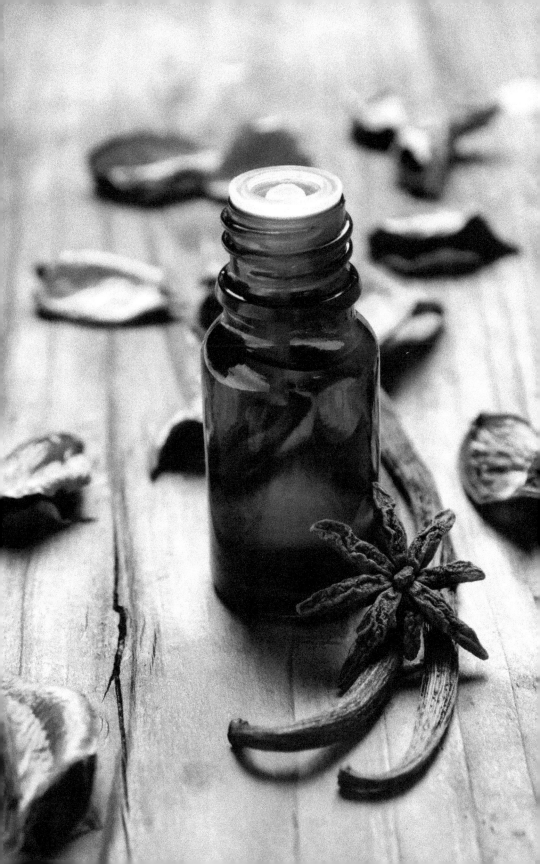

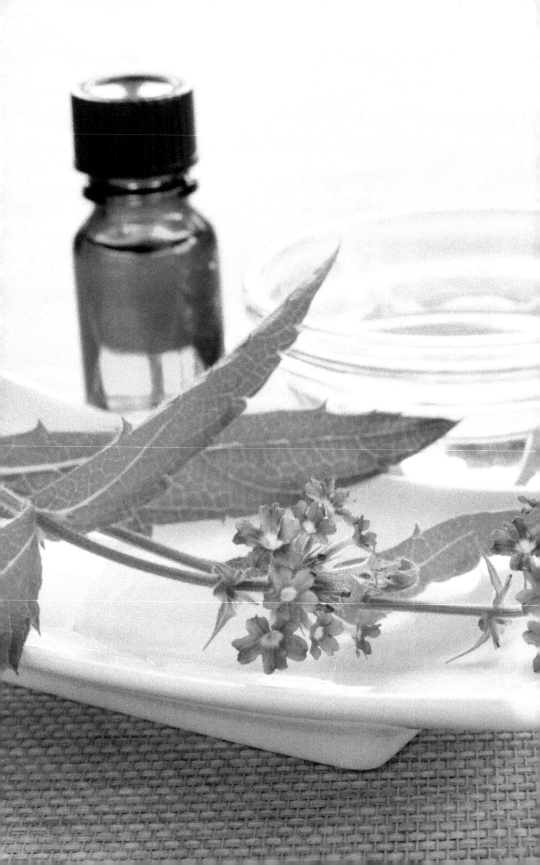

UNDERSTANDING ESSENTIAL OILS

Understanding essential oils is not difficult; in fact, part of their allure is that the methods are quite simple. Albert Einstein—a man who understood how to distill the obscure—once said, "Most of the fundamental ideas of science are essentially simple, and may, as a rule, be expressed in a language comprehensible to everyone."

Although essential oil methods are not complicated, it's important to lay the groundwork and build working knowledge about essential oils, how they are extracted from plants, and what precautions you should take when using them.

By establishing comprehensible language and guidelines, part 1 gives you the tools to freely explore the oils and treatments provided in part 2.

1 LEARN THE BASICS

2 TOOLS FOR SAFE HEALING

3 MASTER THE METHODS

1

LEARN
THE
BASICS

Confidently begin your exploration
of essential oils and their ability to
improve your quality of life

Before you begin experimenting with the healing properties of essential oils, you'll need a basic understanding of
what these substances are and what they can accomplish.
Long before modern humans developed the ability to make
medicines by using chemical synthesis, microbes, hormones, and
enzymes, our ancestors turned to the natural world to find ways
of treating a wide range of ailments. In earlier times, people took
essences from plants and distilled them into oils to soothe pain,
quiet coughs, clear congestion, draw infection out of wounds, and
promote restful sleep. The results they obtained with essential oils
were so good that this ancestral knowledge was passed down to gen-
erations of healers and physicians for thousands of years, first as oral
instructions, then as words written on papyrus and in paper note-
books, and eventually as articles published in professional journals.
In our own time, this information is available online, and essential
oils still qualify as prescription medications in some countries.

Nevertheless, you've probably encountered negative rumors or
disparaging information about essential oils, perhaps online or even
in your doctor's office. This chapter addresses those issues and will
help you begin your exploration of essential oils and their ability to
improve your quality of life. And today, you don't need to distill your
own essential oils. You can purchase them in stores that sell natural
products and promote general health.

WHAT ARE ESSENTIAL OILS?

Essential oils are the true essence of a plant, hence the word *essential*. They come from a group of chemical molecules in plants called terpenes (or hydrocarbons), the cellular-level compounds that create a plant's scent.

*****Terpenes** are organic compounds produced by a plant to create an aroma, a key factor in the plant's ability to protect itself from parasites. Many trees release strong-scented terpenes in warm weather. This process helps create create clouds so that a stand of trees can regulate its own temperature. Terpenes are the main component of essential oils.*

Each plant species has a unique combination of 100 or more terpenes, which make the scent of that species different from the scent of any other. Terpenes may reside in a plant's flowers, roots, leaves, bark, stem, or seeds. Not only do these compounds give plants their powerful scents, they also make plants particularly potent for a wide range of uses—as flavorings in food, as scents and cleaning agents in household and beauty products, and as medicines with demonstrated remedial properties.

Even though we use the term *essential oils*, we are not really talking about oils in their true sense. Think of olive oil, canola oil, almond oil, or sesame oil, for example. What do these oils do when you heat them for cooking? They remain in their liquid state even at high temperatures, which is why they are called fixed oils. But essential oils vaporize when they're heated. That's what makes them easy to inhale in aromatherapy, and it's what makes them effective for other medicinal uses.

*A **fixed oil** is a natural oil that does not change its state when heated. Fixed oils can come from plants or animals, and they usually contain fatty acids, which can be important in a balanced diet.*

HOW ARE ESSENTIAL OILS MADE?

Most essential oils are obtained from plants by one of three basic methods: distillation, expression, and either solvent extraction or hypercritical CO_2 extraction.

Distillation

The first method, distillation, is a process of using steam to break down the plant and capture the compounds within it as they escape in the form of vapor.

Distillation breaks down a plant's leaves, stem, flowers, roots, or bark and captures the terpenes inside.

Distillation begins inside a sealed container, with the plant material placed on a grid to let moisture reach the plant from all sides. The particular distillation method will depend on which parts of the plant contain the terpenes that make up the plant's essence:

- In **water distillation**, the plant is placed in water inside the sealed container, and the water is boiled to produce the steam that breaks the plant down. A distiller will use this method for blossoms, in particular, because water distillation makes it easier for the steam to get through them.
- In **water-and-steam distillation**, the plant stays on mesh above the level of the water so that the steam can move up through the plant.
- In **steam distillation**, there's no water in the container at the beginning of the process. The distiller injects steam into the bottom of the container at high pressure, and the steam rises through the plant matter, softening it so that the essential oil can be obtained.
- In **hydrodiffusion distillation**, the steam enters the container from the top rather than from the bottom. This process creates an environment in which the essential oil can be extracted from tougher parts of the plant, such as the bark, a woody stem, or the seeds.

Once the container has been sealed, the steam—whether produced within the container or injected from outside—softens the plant until the plant's terpenes rise in the form of vapor along with the steam. As the vapor and the steam rise, they travel into a condenser, where they cool until they become two separate liquids—essential oil and water. Then they descend together into a container at the bottom of the condenser, where the essential oil collects on the surface of the water. Because oil and water do not mix, it's fairly easy to siphon off the essential oil.

Expression

The second method of obtaining essential oils is known as expression. This method is used for citrus plants, such as bergamot, lemon, orange, and tangerine.

*Expression, also known as **cold-pressing**, uses a mechanical process to rotate and puncture the rind of a fruit. The essential oil and the juice released from the rind are then collected in a container.*

The juice and oil from citrus fruits were once expressed by hand, but with today's sophisticated equipment, they can both be expressed in massive quantities, with the expressed liquid allowed to stand until the essential oil rises to the top, where it's siphoned off for packaging.

Solvent Extraction and Hypercritical CO_2 Extraction

Specific kinds of essential oils have to be obtained through a third general method, usually because their source plants are too fragile to withstand the deliberate stresses of distillation or expression. One example of this method is solvent extraction, which is used for delicate flowers like jasmine and gardenia. First a solvent is used to draw out the plant's terpenes, its chlorophyll, and some plant tissue as well as the fats or waxes contained in the plant. The substance that results is called a concrete (and has nothing to do with the material used to pave roads). Then the concrete is mixed with alcohol to draw out the scented molecules. The final product of this process is called

ESSENTIAL OILS AND HEALING
A Brief History

....

The use of plants for healing probably began among our earliest ancestors, who determined that certain plants had the ability to help a sick person recover. This information, passed down verbally from one generation to the next, eventually brought about the extraction of essential oils from strong-smelling plants.

Around 1800 BCE, visiting physicians from several Greek and Roman cities arrived in Egypt and left with knowledge about the use of essential oils in healing. In the Bible, nearly 200 mentions of essential oils occur throughout the Old and New Testaments, not the least of which has to do with the three wise men's gift of two plant resins, frankincense and myrrh, to the infant Jesus. Such a gift for a newborn seems absurd from a modern perspective, but these two substances were highly prized for their ability to strengthen a baby's immune system.

The fall of Roman civilization seems to have put much knowledge about essential oils on hold for centuries, but Avicenna, a Persian man of science born in 980 CE, is reputed to have rediscovered the art of distillation, and physicians continued to use essential oils well into the 19th century. Today, researchers at universities around the world are studying essential oils for evidence of their healing properties.

an absolute. Manufacturers of cosmetics and perfumes often use absolutes in their products.

As its name suggests, the method known as **solvent extraction** *uses a solvent—such as methanol, ethanol, hexane, or petroleum ether—to draw the terpenes and other matter out of a plant. The substance that results is called a* **concrete***.*

An **absolute** *is the final product of solvent extraction. It consists of an alcohol-based essential oil extract with about 5 to 10 parts per million (ppm) of solvent residue remaining from the extraction process. Absolutes are normally used only for aromatherapy, but some therapists discourage their use because of these trace amounts of solvents.*

Another example of this third method is known as hypercritical carbon dioxide extraction or CO_2 extraction. This method, which was developed quite recently, makes it possible to capture elements (such as the medicinal properties of plants like frankincense and ginger) that would be lost during one of the more widely used distillation processes. It also produces a more authentic plant fragrance.

Hypercritical CO_2 extraction *uses very high pressure to bring gaseous carbon dioxide to the point where no physical distinction remains between liquid and gas. The dense quasi-liquid that results is able to pass through the plant material and extract the compounds that make up the plant's essential oil. This method is also used to extract caffeine from coffee beans.*

BENEFITS OF ESSENTIAL OILS

Each essential oil has its own properties for healing, relaxation, and mood alteration, and this book provides information about more than 60 of the most popular oils and the benefits you can enjoy from each one. You can use an essential oil to add a few drops of your favorite scent to your bathwater or you can turn to essential oils for aromatherapy. You can add one or more essential oils to your massage oil or you can take advantage of essential oils' medicinal properties. However you use essential oils, you'll find that they're a welcome addition to your personal apothecary.

WHAT IS AROMATHERAPY?

Anytime you use a fragrant plant extract in your bath, as a massage oil, as an inhalant in your home, or for health or healing, you are practicing a form of aromatherapy. The National Association for Holistic Aromatherapy defines this practice as "the art and science of utilizing naturally extracted aromatic essences from plants to balance, harmonize, and promote the health of body, mind, and spirit."[1] An essential oil contains volatile organic compounds extracted from the source plant, and these may be able to improve your health.

Volatile organic compounds (VOCs) are naturally occurring chemicals. Most scents are made up of VOCs. Some VOCs, such as methane, are harmful to the environment, but essential oils are considered to pose far fewer environmental risks.

The essential oils used in aromatherapy may relieve stress or stimulate the body's energy levels. They may promote relaxation and restful sleep. They may also have an effect on depression, high blood pressure, anxiety, chest and nasal congestion, infection, and a wide range of other common ailments. Chapter 4, "A World of Natural Wellness," and appendix A explore essential oils and the many ailments they can be used to treat.

TIPS FOR USING ESSENTIAL OILS

1. **Understand that essential oils are not the same as perfumes.** Most perfumes are made from synthetic ingredients, even when their packaging claims that they are "natural" fragrances. If you're planning to buy an oil for therapeutic purposes, be careful to check the bottle for the words *essential oil.*
2. **Don't shop exclusively by price.** Discount oils may not be as pure as the more expensive ones, and it's also true that the most

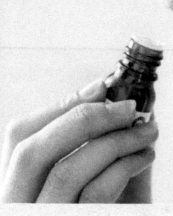

THE SCIENCE OF SCENTS
Essential Oils and Emotion

When you inhale a fragrance, its scent molecules—the VOCs discussed earlier—enter your nose, where they remain in a part of the nasal lining (the olfactory membrane). Within this lining is the olfactory epithelium, a specialized tissue containing receptor neurons (nerve cells) that become containers for the scent molecules.

But these neurons don't just trap the scent molecules and hold them inside the nose. They also send electrical impulses to the brain's olfactory bulb, the center of the sense of smell. The olfactory bulb then signals the amygdala, an area of the brain that contains emotional memories. (This is why the sense of smell is such an immediate trigger for remembering long-ago feelings and events.) The olfactory bulb also distributes signals to the sense of taste, housed in the gustatory center, and this signaling is what makes aromas a key factor in how food tastes.

Olfaction—the sense of smell—is the only one of the five senses that is directly connected to the limbic system, the part of the brain that controls blood pressure, heart rate, and breathing as well as memory and hormone balance. (The other senses—hearing, sight, taste, and touch—are all connected to the thalamus, another region of the brain.) The limbic system regulates fear, anger, depression, anxiety, happiness, and sadness, and it is believed that a scent entering the olfactory bulb has the ability to affect all these emotional responses.

expensive oils are not necessarily the best. A handful of distill-eries sell their essential oils to bottlers all over the world, and so it's entirely possible that all you're buying for a higher price is a fancier label (and a multi-level marketing scheme). See appendix B for a breakdown of essential oil brands.

3. **Remember that essential oils are highly concentrated.** Just a drop or two of most essential oils will be more than enough to produce the desired effect. An essential oil represents a very powerful concentration of terpenes.

4. **Add essential oils to carrier oils.** Because essential oils are so concentrated, they can cause skin irritation and other adverse effects if you apply them directly to your skin. Always dilute your essential oils by adding two or three drops to a carrier oil (a fixed oil like almond oil or grape seed oil) in a ratio of about 50 parts carrier oil to 1 part essential oil. The correct ratios for each essential oil are given in part 2 of this book. Chapter 2, page 26 includes information about the variety of oils that can be used as carrier oils.

*A topically applied essential oil must be mixed with a substance that does not vaporize when exposed to oxygen, the way an essential oil does. That's where a **carrier oil** comes in. As its name suggests, a carrier oil is used to dilute a highly concentrated, potentially irritating essential oil and "carry" it to the skin. Carrier oils come from cold-pressing the fatty parts of a plant, such as the nut, the fruit, or the seed. Many carrier oils (for example, almond oil and grape seed oil) are commonly found in natural foods stores and supermarkets.*

5. **Be aware that essential oils can eat through plastic.** Use only glass bottles with metal lids to store your oils, and only a ceramic or glass bowl to create a blend.

6. **Test your skin for sensitivity before using an essential oil.** It's smart to do a skin test before using an essential oil, just as you would with any kind of topical medication. Add a drop of the essential oil to a teaspoon of a carrier oil or to a cream, wax, or another diluting substance, and then rub a little of the solution on the inside of your upper arm. Wait a few hours and see if

redness or a rash develops. If nothing happens, you're ready to use the diluted oil more liberally. If you do develop redness, you have a sensitivity to this particular essential oil, and you should refrain from using it on your skin.

7. **Not all essential oils are safe for children.** You should rarely use an undiluted essential oil on your own skin, and you should never use one on a child's, because the absorption rate through a child's skin is much faster than through an adult's. For a child, you'll need only half the amount of essential oil recommended for an adult. To be sure that an oil is safe for your child, consult the precautions in chapter 2, "Safety for Babies, Children, and Pregnant Mothers" (page 34) and part 2 of this book. In particular, avoid topical use of lavender oil and tea tree oil on prepubescent boys—these oils' high hormonal-trigger content can cause boys in this age group to grow breasts.[2]

8. **Avoid essential oils during the first trimester of pregnancy, and consider avoiding them throughout your pregnancy.** As you will read over and over in this book, essential oils are natural, but many of them are not recommended for use while you're pregnant—and no essential oil should be used during the first trimester. When you read descriptive information about an essential oil or remedy, look for warnings about pregnancy and nursing.

9. **Treat your essential oils the way you would treat an over-the-counter medication.** Keep them away from children, use them only as directed, and store them in a cool, dry place away from direct sunlight. Many of your essential oils will last for years—the bottle you buy today could still be with you a decade or more from now, and it will retain its full strength. The longevity of an effective essential oil makes that oil a particularly good choice for inclusion in an emergency-preparedness kit.

Notes

1. "What Is Aromatherapy?," National Association for Holistic Aromatherapy, accessed June 23, 2014, http://www.naha.org/explore-aromatherapy/about-aromatherapy/what-is-aromatherapy.

2. "Lavender and Tea Tree Oils May Cause Breast Growth in Boys," National Institutes of Health, US Department of Health and Human Services, *NIH News*, January 31, 2007, http://www.nih.gov/news/pr/jan2007/niehs-31.htm.

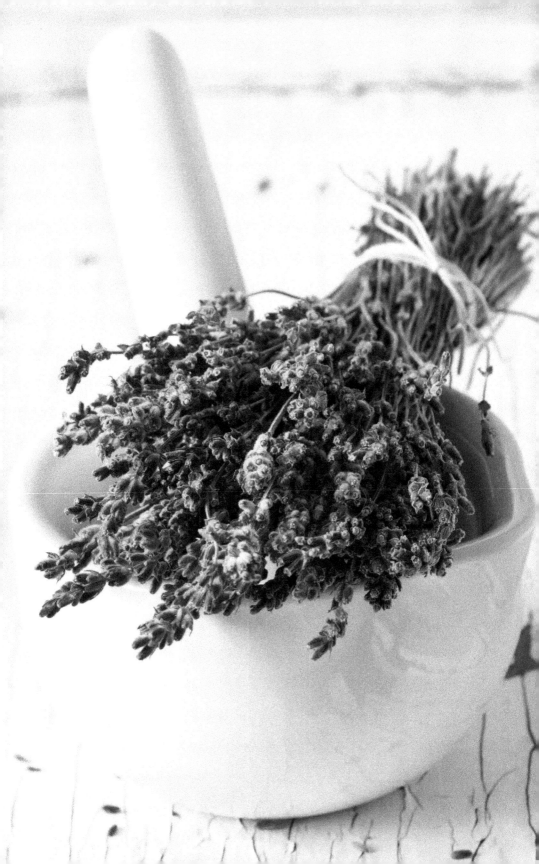

2

TOOLS FOR SAFE HEALING

All you need is the ability to measure
and mix liquids and the patience to
watch for the results you seek

Perhaps you've heard stories from friends or neighbors about the positive effects of using essential oils, or maybe you've talked with your doctor or another health care professional about options for treating common ailments, possibilities that go beyond pharmaceutical medicine. Whatever your current motivation, you've made the decision to learn more about essential oils and their health benefits. Now it's time to start making the most of your determination to find alternatives for you and your family.

It's surprisingly easy to move ahead with essential oils, but it will take some initial setup and a few basic decisions. This chapter provides an overview of the industry, listing names and terms you'll be seeing repeatedly as you become more familiar with the use of oils, and identifying sources you'll use when gathering supplies and tools. The good news is that you don't need any special skills beyond the ability to measure and mix liquids and the patience to wait and watch for the results you seek.

SMART SHOPPING

What is a high-quality essential oil, and how do you know that you're buying one? The buying process can be precarious because there are so many products that claim to be pure or essential when they are not. Sorting through the tricky vocabulary can leave you more confused than informed, so let's begin by clearing up some of the misleading language.

Be very aware of the chain of supply involved in a large part of the essential oils and aromatherapy industry. This industry is not regulated the way the pharmaceutical and food industries are. Almost all essential oils come from only a few distillers around the world, but the companies that buy these distilled oils may either sell them in their purest form or mix them with a variety of additives to increase the volume of particular products. This means that the oil you purchased as "pure" may actually be adulterated. Too many cooks spoil the broth—or, in this case, the oil—so look for essential oils that come to you directly from the distiller. You can purchase these online or through a number of aromatherapy outlets.

. . . .

*The **chain of supply** is made up of all the companies that intervene between the plant growing in the field and the bottle of oil you take home. Growers, distillers, processors, bottlers, distributors, and retailers all have an influence on the product before you buy it.*

*An essential oil is **adulterated** if it contains anything but pure essential oil. If the bottle says that the oil includes a preservative, an alcohol product, or one of many other chemicals, the oil is no longer an essential oil and will not produce the full therapeutic effect you seek.*

. . . .

It's also possible to buy essential oils that are pure but of low quality, either because they were handled or stored improperly or because they came from inferior plants. Low-quality oils are harder to spot because distributors rarely label products as inferior. Your best bet is to do your research and find a distiller or vendor whose products you like and trust. Try purchasing small quantities of one or two essential oils from this distiller or vendor, and see if you get the results you want. Some vendors offer samples of their oils that you can try before making a large purchase. If you are offered this opportunity, take it.

Here are some words to watch for on the labels of commercially available essential oils:

- **Fragrance oil.** This term is used only for oils that are combined with chemicals, or for blends of synthetics. An essential oil will always be called an essential oil.
- **Nature-identical oil.** Any product labeled in this way is not strictly from nature. It may contain extenders or dilutants, two additives that adulterate the oil.

__Extenders__ are additives, either natural or synthetic, that may contain fragrance—chemicals that smell more or less like the essential oil you intended to buy, but that have none of the oil's therapeutic properties. In some cases, extenders are used to make a particularly viscous oil easier to pour.[1]

__Dilutants,__ sometimes called diluents, are colorless, odorless synthetic additives that allow bottlers to stretch the supply of an essential oil. Some dilutants are dangerous for topical use or for use as inhalants, and some may even be carcinogenic.[2]

- **Perfume oil.** Perfumes are made primarily from synthetic compounds, so a product that proclaims itself a perfume is not an essential oil.

- **Pure.** In the absence of official regulation, the word *pure* has become almost meaningless. Many substances that contain chemicals are nevertheless labeled as pure. To get an idea of whether an oil is truly pure, look on the label for the oil's botanical name, country of origin, and method of extraction. If this information is not in evidence, the oil is probably adulterated. In addition, if the label lists any ingredient other than essential oil, the oil is not pure.

- **Synthetic fragrance.** The word *synthetic* on the label says all you need to know.

- **Therapeutic-grade** or **aromatherapy-grade.** These terms have been popularized by multi-level marketing (MLM) companies that sell essential oils. In reality, there is no grading system in the aromatherapy industry, so there is no such thing as a therapeutic-grade or aromatherapy-grade essential oil. (MLM companies, when pressed on this point, claim that these terms reflect their internal standards for quality.)

*In **multi-level marketing (MLM)**, someone who sells a product earns income from her own sales as well as from product sales by the people in her downline, a term referring to those she has recruited into the sales organization. MLM has come under fire from the Federal Trade Commission, which claims that the MLM strategy exploits downline sellers and often amounts to little more than a pyramid scheme.*

The most important thing to remember is that if the label on the bottle does not say *essential oil*, what's inside the bottle is not essential oil (or at least it's not purely essential oil).

Apart from labels, there are several other visual cues that will help you make the best choice when you're in a store and looking at various brands of essential oils:

- **Bulking.** If an essential oil appears to be pure but is markedly less expensive than others of the same variety, it may have been bulked to reduce its cost.

***Bulking** is the practice of extracting essential oils from plants that are from the same species but different harvests, or even using dried plants from previous years along with the current year's fresh plant material. The resulting product is still essential oil, but it may be less effective than a slightly more expensive variety made from a single harvest.*

- **Clear glass bottles.** Essential oils should come in dark glass bottles—usually amber or cobalt—to filter out the ultraviolet (UV) light from the sun and other sources. Oils will deteriorate if they are exposed to direct sunlight or to overhead lighting that includes the UV spectrum.
- **Dusty bottles.** Bottles that have been on the shelf for months or years are likely to gather dust. If a store's essential oils are in dusty bottles, they may have been sitting around for a long time.
- **Loose caps.** Essential oils are volatile, which means that they evaporate when exposed to air. Most evaporate slowly, but if you pick up a bottle in a store and the cap is loose, you may already have lost some of the oil to the air.

- **Rectified, redistilled, folded, or reconstituted oils.** These terms reflect the use of mechanical processes to remove certain natural components from the oils, particularly the terpenes, which create an essential oil's strong scent. The oil products that result are used by the flavoring industry but are not appropriate for aromatherapy or other therapeutic uses. It's unlikely that you will find these oils for sale in stores or on reputable websites where aromatherapy products are sold.

TOOLS AND EQUIPMENT

To use your essential oils effectively, you'll need tools for turning them into inhalants, creams, lotions, and ingestible compounds. You will find a wealth of online sites and places in your community where you can buy the tools you need, and you may be surprised by how much is out there. As you become a more experienced user of essential oils, you'll develop preferences for various tools and equipment, but here are some basic items to get you started.

Must-Haves

- **Bottles and vials.** Once you've discovered a blend of essential oils and a carrier oil that serves a particular purpose, you'll want to mix up a batch, and you'll need a supply of small amber or cobalt glass bottles and vials to hold your favorite concoctions.
- **Cases.** It's important to keep essential oils and blends in a cool, dry place away from direct sunlight—the way you store them will have an impact on their effectiveness over the long term. The aromatherapy industry offers a wide variety of cases in a range of sizes, some as small as a wallet. A case with a lid is the perfect solution to the problem of preserving your oils and keeping them organized in one place at home. But you'll probably want to have several smaller, portable cases, too, so you can keep one filled with your favorite blends in your desk drawer at work and slip another into your suitcase when you're on the road.
- **Diffuser (nebulizer).** This item lets you fill a whole room with the therapeutic aroma of an essential oil or blend. Your diffuser may turn out to be the most important piece of equipment

you'll buy. But don't let yourself get overwhelmed by the large selection of diffusers available for purchase. Start with an inexpensive one, or borrow one from a friend while you're learning how a diffuser works and what type you might like. (For more about diffusers, see chapter 3, page 42.)

- **Droppers.** Sometimes you'll find an essential oil in a bottle that has an orifice reducer, which allows a single drop to be dispensed—a great convenience. Or sometimes an oil comes in a bottle capped with a dropper that has a rubber top. But a dropper like this can be leaky—the last thing you want with an expensive oil. And if the dropper is left in the bottle, the rubber top can deteriorate, ruining the oil and making the bottle unusable. That's why it's best to buy droppers and oils separately (and if you buy a dropper with a rubber top, never leave it in a bottle of essential oil).

- **Funnel.** When the time comes to transfer your blended oils into bottles and vials, you'll be glad you have a funnel. Be sure to choose one that fits your bottles and vials.

- **Pipettes.** Like a dropper, a glass pipette lets you dispense essential oils one drop at a time into carrier oils or lotions. But a pipette can be even better than a dropper—it gives you better control, helps you avoid messy slipups, and eliminates the risk of waste and contamination associated with rubber-topped droppers. These are some of the reasons why many experts in essential oils recommend pipettes over droppers.

- **Syringes.** If you're aiming for high precision when you transfer a measured amount of an essential oil, you'll want to use a syringe. Syringes are marked in increments as small as a drop or a hundredth of a milliliter. This kind of syringe should not be confused with a hypodermic syringe, the kind that has a needle on the end.

Nice-to-Haves

- **Atomizer.** This is the small pump at the top of a perfume bottle. You're going to need an atomizer if you expect to spray your pillow with lavender to promote restful sleep, or if you want to use aromatherapy in this way for other purposes.

- **Blender.** If you plan to combine essential oils with carrier creams and make your own lotions, nothing beats a blender for saving time and effort while getting a thorough mix. You don't have to buy a special or dedicated blender for this purpose, but you also don't want your lotions flavoring your everyday sauces and smoothies. Before and after using your blender to make a lotion, spray the inside with vodka and let it dry or wipe it dry with a clean paper towel.[3] Make sure your blender has a glass jar, not a plastic one.
- **Inhaler.** An inhaler looks like a lipstick case and lets you carry your favorite scent in your pocket or purse. Add a few drops of an oil or blend to the wick inside the inhaler, and take a sniff whenever you need to sharpen your wits, clear your mind, elevate your mood, or fight stress.

Storage

Most essential oils will retain their integrity on the shelf for up to two years, and some will last for up to a decade, as long they're properly stored. You've already learned that you should keep your essential oils in dark-colored glass bottles, away from the sun and other sources of ultraviolet light, so that means no bottles on the kitchen windowsill, no matter how pretty they look. And you know that you can choose from a variety of storage cases. Here are a few more tips for making sure you preserve the full value of your investment in your essential oils:

- **Don't decant oils into plastic bottles.** Essential oils and plastic don't mix. Over time, an essential oil will eat through a plastic bottle. The oil will be ruined, and you'll end up with a mess on your hands.
- **Keep oils away from open flames.** Essential oils are volatile and quick to catch fire, so don't store or use them near a gas stove, a fireplace, or a burning candle.
- **Replace caps tightly.** Just as you need to keep your bottles out of the sun, you need to keep oxygen out of your bottles. You've already been warned that when you're shopping for essential oils in a store, a loose cap on a bottle is a sign that some of the oil

inside has probably evaporated and/or lost potency. A loose cap at home means the same thing—some of your precious oil has vanished into thin air.

- **Store oils in the refrigerator.** You can extend the life of many of your oils, especially citrus oils, by keeping them in the refrigerator. Some oils will solidify in the fridge, but they'll retain their integrity and potency. Just remove them and leave them out long enough to reach room temperature before you use them. The refrigerator is a good place for your carrier oils, too—unlike essential oils, carrier oils grow rancid over time if they're not properly stored.

COMMONLY AVAILABLE CARRIER OILS

It's not unusual for a supplier of essential oils to offer a line of carrier oils, too. As noted in chapter 1, however, many carrier oils are also found in natural foods stores and supermarkets. Although a carrier oil is usually obtained through a cold-pressing or expeller-pressing process that retains the oil's natural color, scent, and constituents, some oils are obtained through maceration.

Constituents *are the parts of a whole oil that are the source of its nutritional or therapeutic value. Suppliers of carrier oils use minimal refining processes to keep the oils from losing their most important parts.*

Maceration *is a process of extracting a plant's essence by soaking plant matter in hot oil and rupturing the cell membranes. The hot oil is then strained to remove the plant matter, then bottled without further processing.*

Unlike cosmetics companies, which refine their carrier oils for more economical use, suppliers of essential oils maintain the integrity of the original oils to maximize the oils' therapeutic value. Here are some of the most common carrier oils, with some tips for choosing what's right for you:

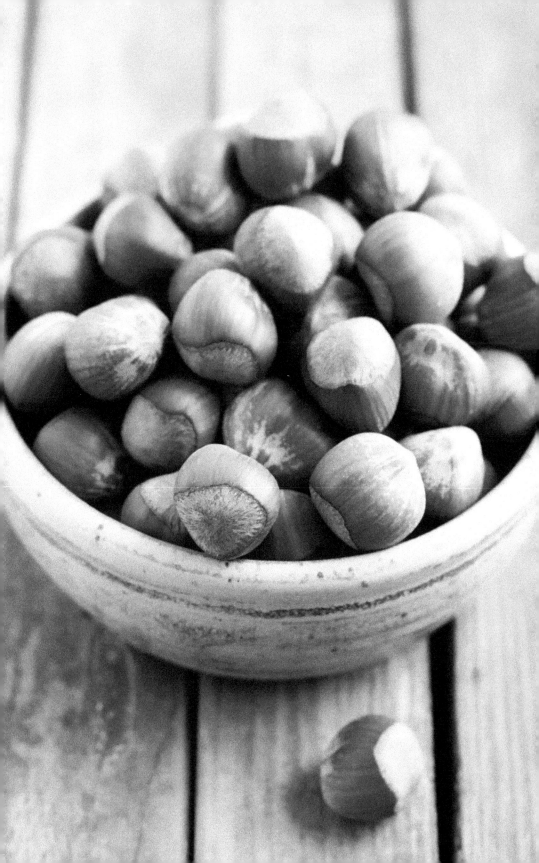

- **Aloe vera oil.** This is one of the great healing oils, providing relief from pain and itching and reducing inflammation. The gelatinous substance that comes from inside the leaves of this succulent plant is collected through maceration of the stems in soybean oil. This substance has long been known as a treatment for first-degree burns and sunburn, so it's not surprising that aloe vera oil can reduce the appearance of scarring. It is even reputed to improve blood circulation.
- **Apricot kernel oil.** A favorite among therapists for facial massage, apricot kernel oil is rich in oleic acid and linoleic acid, two fatty acids that are particularly valued for their ability to revitalize the skin. Apricot kernel oil combines easily with essential oils and spreads smoothly on the skin, properties that could make this your go-to oil for treating acne or slowing down age-related skin changes.
- **Avocado oil.** Rich in vitamins A, D, and E as well as in lecithin and potassium, avocado oil on its own is particularly effective as a remedy for eczema and psoriasis, as a treatment for dehydrated or sun-damaged skin, and as an emollient for skin made dry by the aging process. Avocado oil also mixes well with other carrier oils.
- **Calendula oil.** As a member of the marigold family, the calendula plant produces a large flower resembling a marigold, and it's this flower that is macerated to extract the plant's essence. The carrier oil that results is a versatile treatment for tough wounds like bedsores and skin ulcers, not to mention bruises, varicose veins, burns, diaper rash, eczema, and itching skin.
- **Evening primrose oil.** This oil is extracted from the seeds of the evening primrose plant. It is considered effective against eczema.[4]
- **Grape seed oil.** When you accidentally bite into a grape seed, that astringent taste is exactly what gives grape seed oil its ability to improve skin tone and tighten skin for a more youthful appearance, qualities that make this oil a good choice for facial massage. Grape seed oil can also help clear up acne and is

often used in combination with almond oil and other popular massage oils.

- **Hazelnut oil.** This oil, expressed from the kernels of the hazelnut, has an aroma that is only one of its attributes. Others include its ability to be readily absorbed by the skin, which makes it a good choice for toning and tightening, and its astringent qualities, which make it appropriate for people with oily skin. Its fine texture comes from its high level of unsaturated fats. Hazelnut oil also mixes well with other kinds of oils.

- **Jojoba oil.** When is an oil not an oil? When it's actually a liquid wax that comes from the seed of a plant—in this case, the jojoba plant. Jojoba (pronounced ho-HO-buh) became an important industrial product in the 1970s, after US bans on harvesting whale oil went into effect. Manufacturing companies soon discovered that jojoba was actually superior to whale oil as an additive to cosmetics, and its popularity surged. Jojoba contains myristic acid, which makes it an effective agent for treating inflammation and dry skin. As a carrier oil, it serves as a top-notch moisturizer and often doubles as a hair restorative.

- **Macadamia oil.** This oil contains large amounts of palmitoleic acid, one of the natural oils found on the skin, and serves as an excellent moisturizer. Its emollient properties make it particularly useful for softening aging skin and relieving dryness, and it has so many benefits for the hair that it's used in a number of commercially available conditioners. In catalogs, you may also see it advertised as macademia nut oil.

- **Olive oil.** You're already well acquainted with this oil as a cooking ingredient and a "miracle food" of the Mediterranean diet, but it also has strong medicinal properties. Olive oil, made from the pulp of the olive rather than the kernel, comes in different grades—extra virgin, virgin, and pure—that denote the level of the oil's acidity. Extra-virgin olive oil (popularly known as EVOO) is the highest-quality and most expensive grade, and it contains no more than 0.8 grams of oleic acid per 100 grams of oil. EVOO is pressed mechanically, without the use of solvents.[5] Virgin olive oil contains up to 2 grams of oleic acid per 100 grams

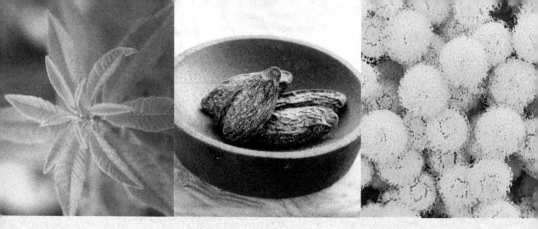

DANGEROUS AND DEADLY
Essential Oils to Avoid

Some essential oils have been banned outright by the Geneva-based International Fragrance Association and are no longer in common use for cosmetics or flavorings, although some are still available for industrial uses.[6] Avoid these oils—some are fatal if swallowed, others are known carcinogens, and still others cause immediate skin sensitization:

- Ajowan
- Balsam of Peru
- Bitter almond
- Boldo leaf
- Cade oil crude
  (prickly juniper)
- Calamus (sweet flag)
- Camphor
- Colophony
- Costusroot (kuth)
- Croton
- Elecampane (scabwort)
- Fig leaf absolute
- Horseradish
- Jaborandi
- Massoia bark
- *Melaleuca bracteata*
- Melilotus

- Mustard
- Ocotea
- Parsley seed
- Rue
- Santolina
- Sassafras
- Savin
- Southernwood
- Styrax gum (oriental
  sweet gum)
- Tansy
- Tea absolute
- Thuja
- Tonka bean
- Verbena
- Wormseed
- Wormwood

of oil. Pure olive oil, a blend of virgin and refined oils, is of lesser quality than EVOO, with a higher level of oleic acid. What this means for you is that EVOO is greener than other grades, a clue that it is the grade of oil closest to the original fruit and most useful as a remedy for inflamed or severely dry skin. But you may find the fragrance of olive oil too close to a food aroma for you to feel comfortable using it as a topical product, and you may also be repelled by its very oily texture.

- **Sesame seed oil.** This oil, expressed from the seed of the sesame plant, smells strongly like a wholesome snack, but if you mix it with almond oil or grape seed oil, you can lighten its heavy, oily texture and somewhat reduce the scent. The moisturizing and emollient properties of sesame seed oil make it a desirable treatment for aging or dry skin, and it has been found effective as a remedy for eczema and other itchy skin conditions.

- **Sweet almond oil.** This oil, obtained from the kernel of the almond, is a favorite with massage therapists because of its pleasant aroma, its soft texture, and its slow rate of absorption through the skin. Sweet almond oil relieves itching and inflammation, promotes a youthful complexion, and contains oleic acids that help nourish the skin. And sweet almond oil can be used by itself—it doesn't need to be combined with any other kind of oil, whether an essential oil or another carrier oil.

- **Walnut oil.** If you're allergic to nuts, be sure to do a skin test before using this oil, since it comes from cold-pressing the nuts of the walnut tree. Walnut oil can be helpful with dry skin but is rarely used alone. There are anecdotal reports of its effectiveness as a balancing agent for the nervous system when used in aromatherapy. Food-grade walnut oil's high antioxidant content has been reported to provide many benefits, including potential resistance to certain kinds of cancer cells.[7]

- **Wheat germ oil.** This oil is made from the wheat plant's germ, or heart, which is rich in protein and minerals. Because its high vitamin E content can prevent rancidity and help lengthen the shelf life of other oils, wheat germ oil is a top choice for mixing with other oils to form a variety of blends. The vitamin E in wheat germ oil also aids the formation and growth of new skin cells, improves circulation, and repairs minor burns, such as sunburn. On its own, however, wheat germ oil is sticky and goopy, a property that makes it a much better mixing oil than a solo choice.

SAFETY CONCERNS

It's easy to confuse what is natural with what is safe, but a number of essential oils are definitely not safe in certain situations. In addition to the issues discussed in "Safety for Babies, Children, and Pregnant Mothers" (page 34) and "Safety for Pets" (page 36), specific cautions should be observed by people who are suffering from or susceptible to the following conditions:

- **Cancer.** Some health professionals recommend that people with cancer avoid aniseed, basil, bay, clove, cinnamon, fennel, ho leaf, laurel, nutmeg, and star anise essential oils. If a cancer is estrogen-dependent, aniseed and star anise essential oils should again be avoided along with citronella, eucalyptus, fennel, lemongrass, and verbena oils.[8] Calamus oil and sassafras oil have been banned from the professional practice of aromatherapy because they contain compounds—asarone and safrole—that have been found to cause cancer. Needless to say, any other substance (such as yellow or brown camphor) that contains either of these carcinogenic compounds should also be avoided. In addition, methyl chavicol, found in some basil oils, may cause cancer when used in large quantities over a period of time.
- **Cardiac (heart) problems.** If you have problems with heart rhythm or blood pressure, avoid using peppermint essential oil, since large amounts of it can increase heart rate and cause palpitations. This book warns against the medically unsupervised oral use of any essential oil, and especially against the ingestion of peppermint oil by anyone who is taking a calcium channel blocker (such as amlodipine) for high blood pressure, since peppermint oil taken by mouth can increase the channel blocker's power.[9] In addition, people with high blood pressure should

avoid using stimulating essential oils, such as hyssop, rosemary, sage, and thyme.[10]

- **Epilepsy.** Some oils are known to have a convulsant effect. People suffering from or at risk for epilepsy or any other convulsive disorder should never use essential oils of camphor, fennel, hyssop, rosemary, sage, or spike lavender (that is, *Lavandula latifolia*, which is not to be confused with normal lavender, or *Lavandula angustifolia*), nor should they use tansy, thuja, or wormwood essential oils.[11]

- **Hepatic (liver) problems.** Essential oils used in massage or aromatherapy are unlikely to have adverse effects on the liver—unless the oils are swallowed, a practice that, again, this book emphatically discourages without the supervision of a knowledgeable physician. Essential oils that can cause liver toxicity if swallowed include aniseed, basil, bay, buchu, cassia, cinnamon, clove, fennel, and tarragon.[12]

- **Sensitive skin.** A large number of essential oils can irritate sensitive skin, even for people who are not officially allergic to the source plants. Other oils can cause phototoxicity—that is, they can increase the skin's sensitivity to the sun (see "Photosensitizing Oils," page 35). If you're interested in using a particular essential oil, check its description in this book so you can avoid using an oil that may leave you vulnerable to phototoxicity, especially on areas of your body that are habitually exposed to the sun. Be sure to perform a skin test, too, as described in chapter 1 (page 15), "Tips for Using Essential Oils."

Special caution is also called for in other situations, and in connection with certain activities:

- **Caring for an elderly and/or frail person.** Before you use any essential oil with someone who is elderly and/or frail, evaluate the precautions associated with the oil against the person's medical conditions to be sure that use of the oil is not contraindicated. Once you're sure it's safe to go ahead, use only half the amount that is normally recommended, since the person's skin may be hypersensitive to substances as well as to the sun.

- **Driving.** You can buy a diffuser that will plug into your car's cigarette lighter and fill your vehicle with scent, but what scent should you choose? Esoteric Oils, an international supplier of essential oils based in South Africa, recommends that you avoid scents that are too relaxing and that induce sleep, such as benzoin, carnation, chamomile, geranium, hops, hyacinth, lavender, linden blossom, mace, marjoram, neroli, nutmeg, ormenis flower, petitgrain, sandalwood, spikenard, valerian, vetiver, and ylang-ylang.[13]

SAFETY FOR BABIES, CHILDREN, AND PREGNANT MOTHERS

Essential oils do come from natural sources, but that doesn't guarantee that they're safe for every person or every use. As noted in chapter 1 (page 16), lavender oil and tea tree oil can cause breast development in prepubescent boys, and a number of essential oils also contain hormones that can adversely affect a baby's development. If you're considering the use of any essential oil for your baby, be sure to check its description in this book, and carefully heed any warnings you find. If you decide to use the oil, measure half the amount (or less) that you would use for yourself, and dilute it with a carrier oil: 1 drop of essential oil in 1 teaspoon of carrier oil.

The same formula applies to older children. When blending massage oil for a child, use half the strength you would use for yourself: a 1 percent dilution instead of the usual 2 percent dilution for an adult (see part 2). And if you're using an essential oil in a diffuser or vaporizer in your child's room, keep the inhalation down to a minute or less, and never leave your child alone with the diffuser or vaporizer, or with any essential oil in any form. Remember, too, that swallowing even a small amount of an essential oil can be very dangerous to a child, so always make sure that your bottles, when not in use, are closed tightly, stored in their case, and placed out of children's reach.

As for the use of essential oils during pregnancy, anecdotal evidence links some oils to spontaneous miscarriage. In fact, some essential oils—including mugwort, parsley seed, pennyroyal, rue, sage, sassafras, savin, thuja, tansy, and wormwood—were used in

PHOTOSENSITIZING OILS
Keep Your Skin Safe

Some plants carry photodynamic agents, molecules that release free radicals and make the skin more susceptible to damaging ultraviolet (UV) rays from the sun and from the UV light found in tanning beds. Oils produced from these plants, especially citrus oils, are very reactive to UV light, and skin to which they have been applied will burn quickly. The skin burns because it has become photosensitized, which is why these are called *photosensitizing oils*. The phototoxicity that occurs is not directly caused by the oils themselves. Instead, it's an effect of the interaction between UV light and the skin to which these oils have been applied.

Be careful with the following essential oils. Don't use them if you expect to be out in the sun within 12 hours of application, and never add any of them to a tanning or sunscreen blend—they won't deepen your tan or protect you from the rays, but they may set you up for the sunburn of your life. Note, however, that the citrus oils marked here with an asterisk—bergamot, bitter orange, grapefruit, lemon, lime, orange, and tangerine (mandarin)—are photosensitizing *only* when they're obtained through cold-pressing, not when they're obtained through steam distillation:

- Angelica
- Bergamot*
- Bitter orange*
- Cumin
- Dill
- Ginger
- Grapefruit*
- Lemon*
- Lemon verbena
- Lime*
- Orange*
- Tagetes
- Tangerine (mandarin)*
- Yuzu

folk medicine specifically as abortifacients (substances capable of inducing an abortion). As you know, this book strongly suggests that you not take any essential oil internally, but these particular oils are especially toxic when swallowed—they can cause multiple organ failure or even death. In addition, *do not use any essential oil during the first trimester.* The hormonal content of some essential oils can disrupt a pregnancy or affect the development of the fetus. Others— angelica, chamomile, cinnamon, clary sage, ginger, jasmine, juniper berry, myrrh, peppermint, rose, rosemary, sweet fennel, and sweet marjoram—can promote menstruation and should obviously be avoided altogether during pregnancy.

In short, if you're not absolutely sure that an essential oil is safe for you, your fetus, your baby, or an older child, follow this simple rule: *Don't use it.*

SAFETY FOR PETS

A few preliminary studies have been conducted in the last few years to determine whether aromatherapy or direct application of essential oils may be good for dogs. But the research remains rudimentary. Veterinarians differ in their experience with and opinions about the effectiveness of essential oils, and even anecdotal evidence is scanty in this area.

Be that as it may, it's never a good idea to leave your essential oils in a place where your dog or cat can get at them. As anyone who lives with a pet knows, an open bottle on a counter is an open invitation to a curious animal. It's well known that dogs have a keen sense of smell. What is less well known is that a cat's sense of smell is even stronger than a dog's. In any case, even a drop of essential oil spilled on a countertop will draw your dog or cat right to the spill, so if you live with a pet, wipe up any oil spills immediately. You should also limit your pet's time in any room where a diffuser is running.

It may turn out that aromatherapy is good for pets—many practitioners have made this claim. But the rest of us need to wait until science has caught up with what is still an open question.

Notes

1. David Crow, "How to Use Essential Oils Effectively: A Comprehensive Overview," Floracopeia, accessed June 26, 2014, www.floracopeia.com/About /how-to-use-essential-oils-effectively.

2. Dorene Petersen, "Quality of Essential Oils: Diluents, Extenders, and Synergy . . . Oh My!," *ACHS Health and Wellness Blog*, December 6, 2013, info.achs.edu/blog /bid/327398/Quality-of-Essential-Oils-Diluents-Extenders-Synergy-Oh-My.

3. Penny Keay, "Aromatherapy Blending and Mixing," Birch Hill Happenings, accessed July 2, 2014, http://birchhillhappenings.com/SE2011blending.htm.

4. "Evening Primrose Oil," University of Maryland Medical Center, last modified June 20, 2013, umm.edu/health/medical/altmed/herb/evening-primrose-oil.

5. "Extra Virgin Olive Oil: What Is Extra Virgin Olive Oil?," *Olive Oil Times*, accessed June 26, 2014, www.oliveoiltimes.com/extra-virgin-olive-oil.

6. "IFRA Banned and Restricted Oils," Esoteric Oils, accessed June 26, 2014, http://www .essentialoils.co.za/banned-oils.htm; see also "Dangerous Essential Oils," Elaine: Webbed, accessed June 26, 2014, http://eethomp.com/AT/dangerous_oils.html.

7. James Heather, "Seven Great Benefits of Walnut Oil," *Medical Daily*, August 4, 2010, www.medicaldaily.com/seven-great-benefits-walnut-oil-231697.

8. "Cancer, Carcinogens, and Essential Oils in Aromatherapy," Esoteric Oils, accessed June 26, 2014, http://www.essentialoils.co.za/cancer.htm.

9. "Peppermint," Heritage Essential Oils, accessed June 26, 2014, http:// heritageessentialoils.com/peppermint.php.

10. "Essential Oil and High Blood Pressure (Hypertension) in Aromatherapy," Esoteric Oils, accessed June 26, 2014, http://www.essentialoils.co.za/high-blood-pressure.htm.

11. "Epilepsy and Essential Oils in Aromatherapy," Esoteric Oils, accessed June 26, 2014, http://www.essentialoils.co.za/epilepsy.htm.

12. "Certain Essential Oils Can Cause Liver Toxicity (Hepatoxicity)," Esoteric Oils, accessed June 26, 2014, http://www.essentialoils.co.za/liver-toxicity.htm.

13. "Essential Oils to Avoid When You Need to Concentrate," Esoteric Oils, accessed June 26, 2014, http://www.essentialoils.co.za/concentration.htm.

3

MASTER
THE
METHODS

With regular practice, you'll soon get
the hang of measuring, dispensing,
and blending essential oils

This chapter tells you everything you need to know about aromatic and topical methods of using essential oils (as explained earlier, this book is not a guide to internal use). You'll probably need some time to get the hang of measuring, dispensing, blending, and mixing essential oils. But with regular practice, the preparation process will become second nature.

AROMATIC METHODS

Your sense of smell will be pleasantly engaged by the aromatic methods of using essential oils. Whether you're inhaling an oil right from the bottle, sniffing an oil-infused cotton ball, or using an oil in a humidifier, a vaporizer, a diffuser, a nebulizer, or a facial steamer, don't be deceived by those gentle, lovely aromas—essential oils pack a serious therapeutic punch.

Essential Oils for Direct and Indirect Inhalation

What could be simpler than removing the cap from a bottle of essential oil and breathing in the oil's aroma? With this method, known as *direct inhalation*, you get the oil's beneficial effects immediately, whether you're seeking to sharpen your concentration with peppermint, myrrh, sandalwood, or frankincense oil, or boost your immune system with thyme oil, or calm your nerves with chamomile oil.

When you use the method known as *indirect inhalation*, you apply undiluted essential oil to a piece of fabric, a cotton ball, a shirt collar, or a pillow case—a practice known as using the oil *neat*—or you place the oil in a heating or air conditioning duct or use a cotton ball to dab it on the slats of a car's air vents.

A LITTLE GOES A LONG WAY

You may be accustomed to thinking that if a small amount of something is good, a large amount must be even better, but that's not the way essential oils work. In fact, using them that way can be hazardous to your health. Remember, essential oils are highly concentrated, so they're used in very small quantities, and most often they're diluted with carrier oils or creams. Chapter 8 includes information about essential oils that are potential skin irritants.

WHAT TO DO

For direct inhalation, hold an uncapped bottle of essential oil close to your nose and take a few deep breaths, or place a few drops of the oil on a cotton ball and inhale three or four times. For indirect inhalation, apply the undiluted essential oil to fabric or cotton right from the bottle.

WHAT TO WATCH OUT FOR

One distributor of essential oils, dōTerra Aromatics, suggests placing a few drops of an essential oil on your palm, rubbing your hands together, holding your hands over your face, and inhaling.[1] If you follow this suggestion, take care to avoid getting the oil in your eyes—that would cause you significant discomfort—and perform a skin patch test first (see chapter 1, page 15). Always pay attention to how your body reacts to any essential oil to make sure you're not overusing the oil or having a bad reaction. Chapter 8 includes information about possible adverse reactions to essential oils.

Essential Oils in a Humidifier

A humidifier keeps the air in a room moist by dispersing a fine cool mist or releasing puffs of steam. This device can relieve dry skin as well as dryness of the mouth and nasal passages, especially in desert climates or areas where winters are cold and dry. A humidifier can also alleviate symptoms of a cold or the flu, and when it's used with an essential oil, it can even improve your mood and sharpen your mind.

WHAT TO DO

Open your humidifier's water chamber, which is just what it sounds like—the part of the humidifier where the water goes. After you've filled the chamber to the specified level, add the recommended number of drops of essential oil (usually between 3 and 9), and turn the humidifier on.

WHAT TO WATCH OUT FOR

In general, children should not handle humidifiers, and no child should ever be left alone in a room with a humidifier that heats water to release steam. Don't allow a humidifier to spray mist onto a wall, either—the wall can become saturated, and the moisture can turn to mold. To prevent mold from developing inside a humidifier, rinse the device out and dry it after each use.

Essential Oils in a Vaporizer

A vaporizer is essentially a humidifier that has a single purpose—to release warm, comforting steam. Vaporizers designed for use with essential oils often have two chambers, one for the water and one for a heat source, whether that's a candle or an electrical heating element. Some also include what's called a *medicine well*, or cup, which rests above the water and holds the essential oil.

WHAT TO DO

Fill the vaporizer's water chamber to the specified level, and either add 6 to 8 drops of essential oil to the water or place the oil in the medicine well. Then turn the vaporizer on. If you live in a hard-water area, you may want to pick up some demineralizing tablets from a pharmacy and add them to the water to keep mineral deposits from collecting inside the vaporizer and shortening its life.

All the same precautions that apply to a humidifier should be observed with a vaporizer, but you need to be extra careful if your vaporizer uses a candle to heat the water.

Essential Oils in a Diffuser

Like a humidifier, a diffuser creates mist and sends it into the air, but a diffuser has no heating element. Hundreds of different styles are available for use with essential oils, to scent your environment, help you focus or relax, change your mood, and even boost your immune system. Some diffusers have an automatic shutoff, some feature a remote control or lights, and some even play relaxing music, although you may not need all those extras. Look for a diffuser that runs quietly, is easy to clean, and either has no light or has one that you can turn off if you want to use your diffuser overnight. You will also want a diffuser that can produce mist for a large area, such as the entire first floor of your house.

WHAT TO DO

Fill the diffuser's reservoir with filtered or distilled water, and add 8 to 15 drops of essential oil. If you just want to enjoy the scent, run the diffuser for 15 to 30 minutes, the period during which your nose can still discern the fragrance. For therapeutic use, run the diffuser beyond your nose's ability to detect the scent. To switch fragrances midstream, so to speak, transfer the scented water in the diffuser to a ceramic or glass container (so you can use it again later) and then dry the reservoir with a towel, refill it with fresh water, and add 8 to 15 drops of a different oil.

WHAT TO WATCH OUT FOR

Because a diffuser has no heating element, it's safer around children than a vaporizer, but it's always crucial to make sure kids and pets don't have access to water containing essential oils.

HOW BIG IS A DROP?

Throughout this book, you'll find instructions for using essential oils according to recipes that call for specific numbers of drops. But how much oil do you need for 2 or 5 or 8 drops? This table will help you keep your measurements precise and your remedies safe and effective.

Drops	Milliliters (ml)	Percentage (%) of 1 Ounce*
6	0.30 ml	1.0
12	0.60 ml	2.0
15	0.75 ml	2.5
30	1.50 ml	5.0
60	3.00 ml	10.0

* 1 ounce = 600 drops (30 ml)

Source: Adapted from "Methods of Application," Nature's Gift, http://www.naturesgift.com/methods.htm

Essential Oils in a Nebulizer

In physician-supervised respiratory therapy, a nebulizer is a device that uses compressed air to deliver medication directly into a patient's bronchial tubes and lungs for a short time by way of a mask that fits over the patient's nose and mouth. The type of nebulizer used in aromatherapy doesn't include a mask. Instead, it converts essential oil into a fine mist of microparticles and releases them into the air through a spout, perhaps over a period of several hours. Peppermint essential oil is a popular one for use in nebulizers. This oil is often used to promote alertness and is even said to increase pain tolerance.[2]

THE DO-IT-YOURSELF DIFFUSER

Want the benefits of a diffuser without the price tag of a fancy device? Just put the kettle on, boil some water, let the boiled water cool a bit, pour it into a glass or ceramic bowl, add 10 to 20 drops of an essential oil or oil blend, and place the bowl of scented water wherever you want to enjoy its pleasant or therapeutic effects.

WHAT TO DO

Place a few drops of essential oil in the nebulizer's well, and turn the device on. When all the oil has been used up and no more vapor is being released from the nebulizer, turn the device off and clean it thoroughly.

WHAT TO WATCH OUT FOR

Do not use a nebulizer with a mask and never directly inhale the microparticles of essential oil released by a nebulizer. Doing so can irritate your bronchial tubes and lungs and even cause a toxic reaction. It's best not to use a nebulizer with plastic parts, since essential oils can eat through plastic.

Essential Oils in a Facial Steamer

This device heats water at high pressure and delivers a steady infusion of steam right to your face, hydrating your skin and extracting impurities while preserving your complexion.

WHAT TO DO

Fill the steamer's reservoir with distilled or filtered water (or tap water, if your steamer is made to use it). Put 8 to 15 drops of your essential oil or blend in the receptacle provided for it, usually near the device's steam vent. (Some steamers require the oil to be applied to a cotton ball or cloth, which is then placed in the receptacle.) Turn the device on and let it heat up and start producing steam. Use the device's nozzle to direct the steam toward the area you want to treat.

WHAT TO WATCH OUT FOR

Steam can burn your skin, so pay attention, and don't overuse your steamer.

TOPICAL METHODS

Although massage is probably the best-known topical use of essential oils, they're also used topically in acupuncture and acupressure, in hot compresses and cold packs, in bathing and showering, and sometimes in direct application to the skin.

Essential Oils for Massage

In massage, an essential oil is diluted with a single carrier oil or a blend of several carrier oils before being applied to the skin. The person receiving the massage benefits from the oil's absorption into the skin as well as from the release of the oil's aroma into the air.

WHAT TO DO

See "Mixing Oils for Massage," page 47.

WHAT TO WATCH OUT FOR

If you're blending a massage oil for use with a child, reduce the dilution from 2 percent to 1 percent (see "How Big Is a Drop?," page 43). With children as well as adults, avoid using any essential oil known to be a skin irritant (see chapter 8).

Essential Oils in Acupuncture and Acupressure

Many practitioners of acupuncture and acupressure are also experts in herbal therapy, and recently they've begun to incorporate the essential oils into their work. For example, the points of acupuncture needles can be swabbed with one or more diluted oils or blends, and dilutions of essential oils and blends can be applied directly to the skin at the acupressure points associated with particular ailments. Essential oils combined with acupuncture and acupressure can reduce stress, boost immunity, increase vitality, help relieve pain, reduce the discomforts of menstruation and menopause, clear up skin issues, and promote wellness in other areas.

WHAT TO DO

If you're seeing a practitioner of acupuncture or acupressure, ask about using essential oils to support your wellness goals.

WHAT TO WATCH OUT FOR

Be sure to tell your practitioner about any skin sensitivities, allergies, or other adverse reactions you've experienced in your own work with essential oils.

Essential Oils in Warm Compresses and Cold Packs

If you have a muscle injury, a wound, or arthritis pain, adding essential oil to a warm compress can increase the known benefits of heat, moisture, and gentle pressure. This treatment can also relieve menstrual cramps, stomachache, intestinal cramping, boils, toothache, and chronic pain from old injuries. The benefits of a cold pack—pain relief for injuries along with reduction of swelling and inflammation—can be enhanced by the healing properties of essential oils.

WHAT TO DO

See "How to Make a Warm Compress," page 48. Follow the same instructions to make a cold pack, but use refrigerated water or an ice bath (ice mixed with water) instead of hot water.

WHAT TO WATCH OUT FOR

Always be sure to dilute your essential oils. For a hot compress, never use water hot enough to burn your skin. If you're using a cold pack, be aware that ice placed directly on the skin can cause numbness

MIXING OILS FOR MASSAGE
Enhance the Sense of Relief

....

1. When you use essential oils to make your own massage oils or lotions, use a 2 percent dilution in a carrier oil (see "How Big Is a Drop?," page 43). That may seem like a very weak concentration if you're accustomed to strongly scented commercial shampoos, hand soaps, body sprays, and other products, but it's all you need for the effects of an essential oil to be experienced.

2. Use only carrier oils that are 100 percent natural. Synthetic carrier oils can block the effects of essential oils. To boost the effects of massage with essential oils, choose carrier oils that have therapeutic properties of their own (see chapter 2).

3. Combine essential oils with carrier oils by gently mixing them in a small ceramic or glass bowl. If you're combining an essential oil with a thicker lotion, butter, or cream, you may want to use a blender (see chapter 2).

4. After a massage with essential oils, there's no need to shower. Allow the oils to be absorbed slowly.

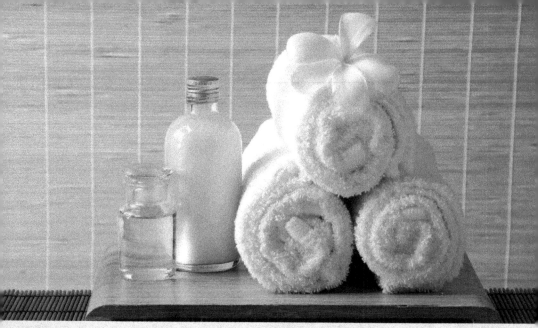

HOW TO MAKE
A WARM COMPRESS
Heal with Heat

1. Fill a basin (not made of plastic) with about a pint of water as hot as you can comfortably stand.
2. Add 3 or 4 drops of your selected essential oil. If you're using more than one type of essential oil, add no more than 4 drops total.
3. For your compress, choose a hand towel, another small piece of fabric, or a cloth bandage.
4. Place the compress on the surface of the water, and let the compress become completely saturated.
5. Lift the compress from the bowl of water, and wring out any excess.
6. Place the wet compress on the area to be treated. To contain the moisture, cover the compress with a plastic bag or a sheet of plastic wrap, and hold the compress and the plastic in place with a towel or an elastic bandage wrapped just tightly enough to keep the compress from slipping.
7. When the compress cools to body temperature, replace it with another warm compress.

and even frostbite, so remove the cold pack right away if the numbness develops in the area being treated.

Essential Oils for Bathing and Showering

Adding one or more essential oils to a bath is an easy way of enjoying their benefits, both as you inhale them and as they make contact with your skin. Bathing with properly diluted essential oils can relax you, promote good circulation, soothe your skin, and relieve respiratory ailments and muscle aches as well as premenstrual syndrome and menstrual cramps.

In the shower, combine your chosen essential oils with an unscented body wash, or with sugar or salt to create an invigorating scrub that delivers the oils' benefits right to your skin. At the very least, this approach will help relieve such skin conditions as dryness and loss of elasticity. Any broader benefits will be determined by the essential oils you choose.

WHAT TO DO

To prevent essential oils from simply floating on top of your bathwater and potentially irritating your skin, add 5 to 10 drops of your essential oil or essential oil blend to half a cup of bath salts, milk, or sesame oil, and then pour that mixture into your bath. (See chapter 4, page 142, for instructions on making your own bath salts.)

For a shower, add 5 drops of your chosen essential oil for each ounce of liquid body wash. Be sure to blend the oil completely with the wash before applying the mixture to your skin. If you're using a sugar scrub, thoroughly combine 1 cup of sugar, ½ cup of a carrier oil, and 8 drops of your selected essential oil. Apply the mixture in the shower, and rinse it off thoroughly.

WHAT TO WATCH OUT FOR

Some essential oils can be irritants and should not be added to bathwater or mixed with a liquid body wash or with sugar or salt. They include cinnamon, clove, lemongrass, oregano, thyme, and cold-pressed bergamot, bitter orange, grapefruit, lemon, lime, orange, and tangerine/mandarin oils.

Essential Oils for Layering

Layering is direct application of one essential oil to the skin, followed several minutes later by direct application of a second essential oil. This method is considered to be potentially more effective than the use of a blend, since each oil is used at full strength. It also allows the pairing of two oils that may not be available in a commercial blend.

WHAT TO DO

Place a drop of the first oil directly onto your skin, rub the oil to distribute it over the area being treated, wait about six minutes, and repeat the procedure with a drop of the second oil, applied to the same place and rubbed for distribution over the first oil. Use two oils that have similar properties—for example, two antibacterial oils or two antifungal oils. You may also choose to use a single oil for one layer and a blend containing that oil for the other layer. Bear in mind that the two oils you choose for layering may have clashing scents, so hold the two bottles under your nose to determine how they smell together before you layer them.

WHAT TO WATCH OUT FOR

Before you begin, check chapter 8 to determine if the essential oil you want to use is safe to use directly on skin. Be sure to perform a skin patch test with each of the oils you intend to use (see chapter 1, page 15).

Notes

1. "Direct Inhalation of Essential Oils in Aromatherapy," dōTerra Aromatics, accessed July 2, 2014, www.doterra-aromatics.com/info/inhalation.html.

2. Laurice Maruek, "Peppermint Oil in a Nebulizer," LiveStrong, August 16, 2013, www.livestrong.com/article/222093-peppermint-oil-in-a-nebulizer.

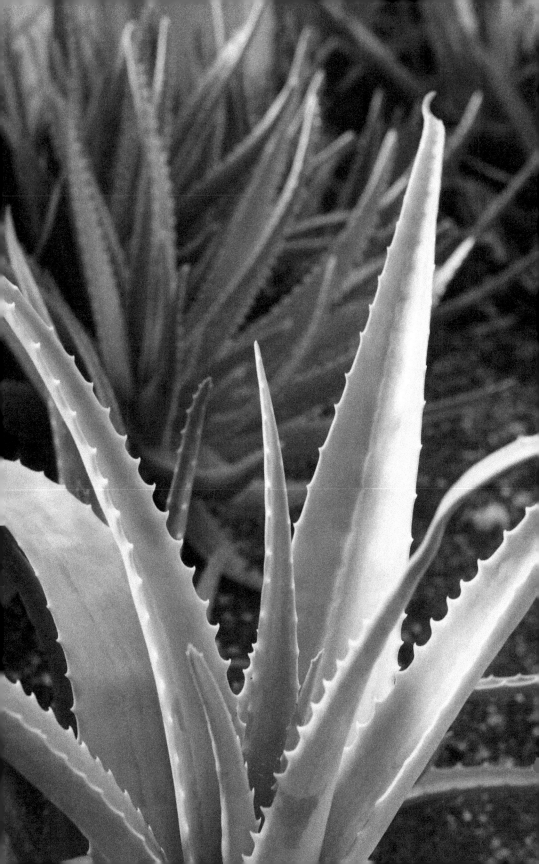

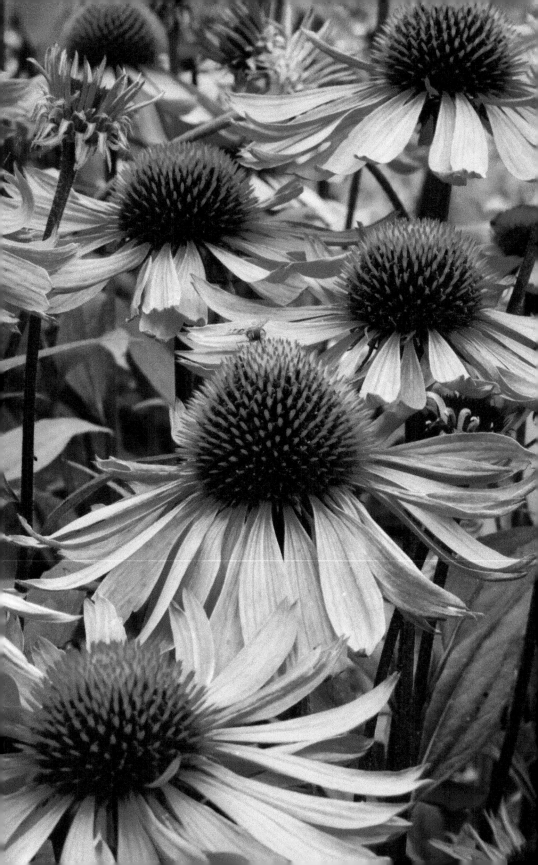

NATURE'S PRESCRIPTIONS

Whether you're looking for a natural way to shorten a cold or a method for fading freckles, you'll find the remedy you seek in the following pages. Essential oils can become your go-to solutions for health and wellness, your natural beauty regimen, your chemical-free clean house, or a way to bring a breath of spring into your home in the dead of winter. You'll also find information to help you build your personal apothecary of essential oils, so you can be ready for any illness, condition, or cleaning day.

4 A WORLD OF NATURAL WELLNESS

5 WELLNESS AND BEAUTY BOOSTS

6 SIMPLE SCENTS AND PLEASURES

7 YOUR NATURAL HOME

8 YOUR PERSONAL APOTHECARY

4

A WORLD OF NATURAL WELLNESS

Essential oils are effective against
dozens of ailments, from acid reflux
to whooping cough

N ow that you have a basic understanding of how to use essential oils, it's time to put your new knowledge to work. This chapter tells you which oils are effective against dozens of ailments, from acid reflux to whooping cough, and gives you instructions for making your own remedies.

The remedies that follow have been selected carefully for their documented effectiveness and their basis in science. At universities around the world, research has proved that some essential oils are as effective as pharmaceuticals in relieving symptoms and promoting wellness. Not all essential oils have been tested in laboratories, however, and many have been tested only in labs and not on human beings. Use your best judgment in choosing the remedies that are right for you and your family.

Essential oils are not a substitute for medical care. In all cases, these remedies should be used alongside a medical approach—especially for chronic conditions (asthma, colitis, depression, diabetes, and heart disease, for example)—and not in lieu of a doctor's care. Talk to your doctor before using any essential oil to be sure it will not react with a medication you are already taking. If your condition gets worse, seek medical help as soon as possible.

Acid Reflux

When acidic digestive juices in the stomach back up into the esophagus, the result can be a painful level of discomfort known as *heartburn* (because of the burning sensation) or *acid reflux*.

RUB

1 teaspoon carrier oil
4 or 5 drops frankincense essential oil

1. Pour the carrier oil into a small glass or ceramic bowl.
2. Add the frankincense essential oil to the carrier oil, and stir to combine.
3. At bedtime, rub this blend on the stomach, throat, and chest.

Acne

Acne is a skin condition aggravated by hormonal changes. Essential oils can help clear up blemishes and prevent the formation of new ones by cleansing the skin and fighting the production of sebum, the oily substance that can clog pores.

NEAT TREATMENT

3 or 4 drops tea tree essential oil

1. Transfer the tea tree essential oil to a small glass or ceramic bowl.
2. Using a cotton swab, apply the undiluted tea tree essential oil directly to blemishes.

IT'S MORE THAN ACADEMIC Two clinical studies, one from 1990 and the other from 2007, have confirmed tea tree oil as an effective treatment for acne.[1]

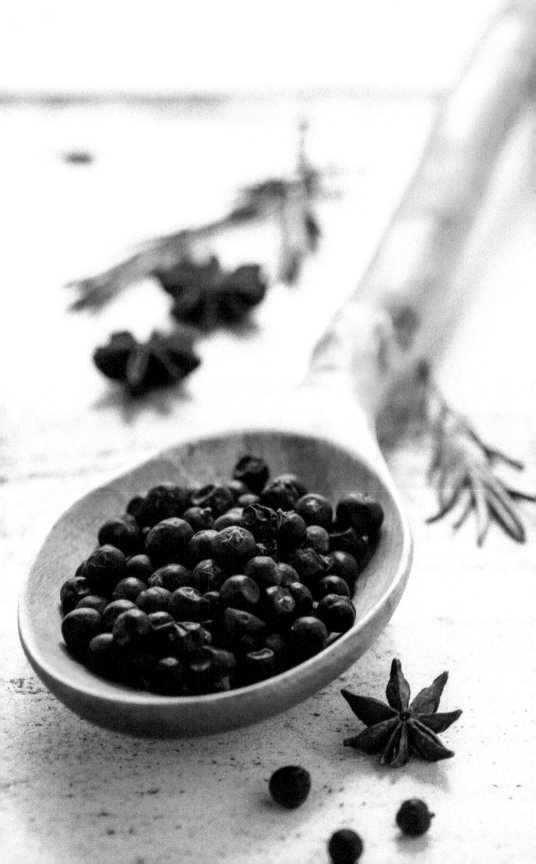

MASK

To make a base powder for the mask

2 ounces green clay (available in powdered form
    at natural foods stores)
3 teaspoons corn flour

1. Mix the clay with the corn flour to create the mask powder.
2. Store the powder in a covered jar until you're ready to use it.

To make and use the mask

1 tablespoon mask powder
1 tablespoon brewer's yeast
1 tablespoon water
1 drop juniper berry essential oil
1 drop lavender essential oil

1. Mix the mask powder with the brewer's yeast in a glass or
   ceramic bowl.
2. Add the water to form a paste.
3. Add the juniper berry and lavender essential oils, and stir
   to combine.
4. Apply the mixture to the face, and leave it on for 15 minutes,
   then rinse and pat dry.

STEAM TREATMENT

3 cups hot water
1 drop clary sage essential oil
1 drop thyme essential oil

1. Pour the hot water into a glass or ceramic bowl.
2. Add the clary sage and thyme essential oils (they will remain on
   the water's surface).
3. Drape a towel over your head in such a way that it is also draped
   closely over the bowl.
4. Bend to hold your face over the bowl. *Keep your eyes closed.*

5. Remain in this position for about 5 minutes, periodically lifting one side of the towel to take a breath of fresh air.
6. After 5 minutes, sit back up and remove the towel.
7. Rinse your face with cold water to close the pores.

NEAT BEDTIME BLEND

30 drops orange seed essential oil
15 drops carrot essential oil
3 drops chamomile essential oil

1. Transfer the orange seed, carrot, and chamomile essential oils to a dark-colored glass bottle that closes tightly.
2. At bedtime, using a cotton ball, apply 5 drops of this undiluted blend to skin affected by acne.
3. Leave the blend on for 5 minutes.
4. After 5 minutes, use a tissue to remove any excess oil.
5. Repeat this treatment once a day at bedtime until the acne fades.

EARLY-WARNING DAB-ON BLEND

1 teaspoon jojoba or coconut carrier oil
3 drops oregano essential oil

1. Pour the jojoba carrier oil into a small glass or ceramic bowl.
2. Add the oregano essential oil to the carrier oil.
3. Using a cotton ball, dab this blend on skin where acne is about to appear, as indicated by the appearance of spots that characteristically precede an outbreak.
4. Repeat this treatment once a day until the spots are gone.

Age Spots

What used to be called *liver spots* (since they were once believed to have something to do with liver function) are small and generally harmless tan, brown, or black spots on the skin where pigmented cells have clumped together. You may choose to have a dermatologist remove your age spots, but the following remedies can help fade them.

¼ cup coconut carrier oil

6 drops frankincense essential oil

6 drops lavender essential oil

6 drops myrrh essential oil

To make the blend

1. Put the coconut carrier oil in a glass or ceramic cup.
2. Add the frankincense, lavender, and myrrh essential oils to the carrier oil, and stir to combine.
3. Pour the blend into a dark-colored glass bottle that closes tightly, and store the bottle in the refrigerator between uses.

To use the blend

1. Using a cotton ball, apply this blend once a day to skin affected by age spots.
2. Repeat this treatment for several weeks, or until you notice results.

TWICE-A-DAY BLEND

1 ounce organic castor oil

10 drops frankincense essential oil

To make the blend

1. Pour the castor oil into a small glass or ceramic bowl.
2. Add the frankincense essential oil to the castor oil, and stir to combine.
3. Pour the blend into a dark-colored glass bottle that closes tightly, and store the bottle in the refrigerator between uses.

To use the blend

1. Using a cotton ball, apply this blend to skin affected by age spots.
2. Repeat this treatment 2 times a day for 4 weeks, or until you notice results.

20 drops avocado carrier oil

6 drops sandalwood essential oil

4 drops blue cypress essential oil

4 drops lavender essential oil

4 drops nutmeg essential oil

To make the blend

1. Pour the avocado carrier oil into a small glass or ceramic bowl.
2. Add the sandalwood, blue cypress, lavender, and nutmeg essential oils to the carrier oil, and stir to combine.
3. Pour the blend into a dark-colored glass bottle that closes tightly, and store the bottle in the refrigerator between uses.

To use the blend

1. Using a cotton ball, apply 2 to 4 drops to skin affected by age spots.
2. Repeat this treatment 3 times a day for 2 weeks.

Aging Skin

Skin changes happen for all of us as we grow older. Here are some natural ways to help mature skin maintain its purity, tone, and firmness.

CLEANSING PASTE

4 ounces almonds

3 ounces sweet almond carrier oil

2 ounces apple cider vinegar

2 ounces spring water

6 drops essential oil (good choices: bois de rose, borage seed, carrot, evening primrose, galbanum, lavender, myrrh, neroli, rose, or violet leaf)

To make the blend

1. Grind the almonds in the glass jar of a blender.
2. Add the sweet almond carrier oil, apple cider vinegar, spring water, and essential oil to the ground almonds.
3. Blend the ingredients on high for at least 2 minutes to produce a smooth paste.

To use the blend

1. Using a soft, natural-bristle complexion brush, apply the paste to your face.
2. After 30 seconds, rinse your face with cool water to remove the paste.[2]

TONING BLEND

½ cup white wine
10 drops rosemary essential oil
3 drops peppermint essential oil

To make the blend

1. In a small saucepan, simmer the wine for 10 minutes.
2. Let the wine cool until tepid.
3. Pour the wine into a heatproof glass or ceramic bowl.
4. Add the rosemary and peppermint essential oils to the wine, and stir to combine.
5. Pour the mixture into a 4-ounce dark-colored glass bottle that closes tightly, and store the bottle in the refrigerator between uses.

To use the blend

1. Using a cotton ball, smooth the toner over your face.
2. Use the toner within 6 months.

MOISTURIZING BLEND

½ cup olive carrier oil
¼ cup apricot kernel carrier oil

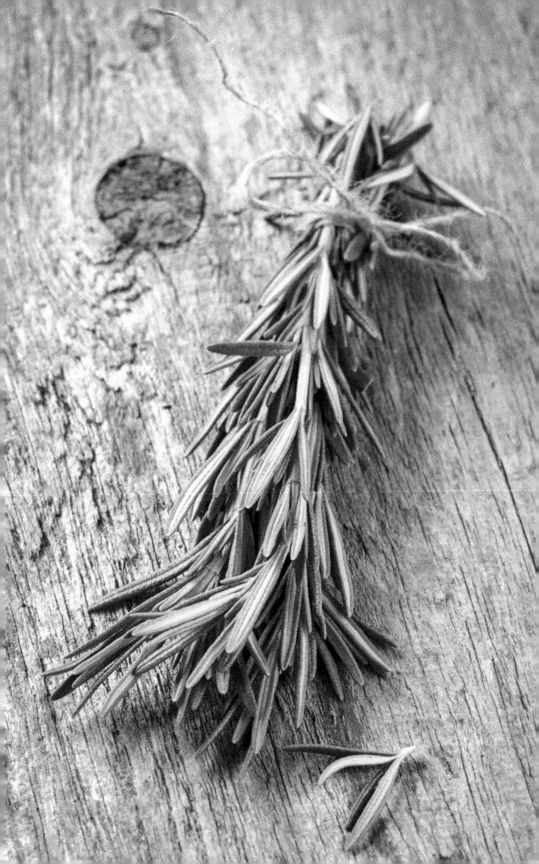

30 drops carrot seed essential oil

20 drops rose hip seed essential oil

To make the blend

1. Pour the olive and apricot kernel carrier oils into a glass or ceramic bowl.
2. Add the carrot seed and rose hip seed essential oils to the carrier oils.
3. Pour this blend into a 6-ounce dark-colored glass bottle that closes tightly, and store the bottle in the refrigerator between uses.

To use the blend

Using your fingertips, gently apply a small quantity of the blend to your face and neck once a day.

Allergies (Seasonal)

In the United States alone, more than 60 million people experience seasonal allergies. There are over-the-counter medications that do a good job of treating the symptoms, but at the cost of side effects that include dry mouth, drowsiness, and other discomforts. As an alternative, try these natural remedies.

DIFFUSER TREATMENT

8 to 15 drops lavender essential oil

1. Add the lavender essential oil to the water in your diffuser.
2. Turn the diffuser on, and let it run for 15 minutes every 2 hours.
3. For continuous treatment, place the diffuser next to your bed, and let it run all night.

½ teaspoon olive carrier oil
2 drops peppermint essential oil

1. Pour the olive carrier oil into a small glass or ceramic bowl.
2. Add the peppermint essential oil to the olive oil, and stir to combine.
3. Using a cotton ball, dab the oil around your nostrils.

DON'T BE A NEAT FREAK Be sure to dilute peppermint essential oil if you're dabbing it around your nose to relieve allergy symptoms. If you use the oil neat, it will make the inflamed skin burn.

Anemia

A shortage of hemoglobin (healthy red blood cells) is a medical condition that may have a number of causes, including chronic or internal bleeding. Once your doctor has ruled out a serious illness as the source of the deficiency, anemia can be treated fairly reliably with changes in diet and the addition of nutritional supplements. Essential oils will be absorbed into your skin and can also help strengthen the production of red blood cells.

NEAT TREATMENT

1 drop helichrysum, lemon, or lemongrass essential oil

Using a cotton ball, apply the undiluted helichrysum essential oil to the soles of your feet and the inside of your wrists.

NEAT BLEND

1 drop helichrysum essential oil
1 drop lemon essential oil
1 drop lemongrass oil

1. Add the helichrysum, lemon, and lemongrass essential oils in a small glass or ceramic bowl, and stir to combine.
2. Using cotton ball, apply the undiluted blend to the soles of your feet and the inside of your wrists.

Anxiety

Aromatherapy can be very effective with the anxiety that accompanies current happenings as well as thoughts about future circumstances and events. Several essential oils can help restore your sense of well-being if you get knocked off balance after interacting with coworkers or family members, or if you need to meet several important goals all at the same time.

DIFFUSER TREATMENT

8 to 15 drops essential oil (good choices: bergamot, chamomile, Douglas fir, rose otto, or sandalwood)

1. Add the essential oil to the water in your diffuser.
2. Turn the diffuser on, and let it run for at least 15 minutes.

BATH BLEND

½ cup milk
4 drops sandalwood essential oil
1 drop ylang-ylang essential oil

1. Pour the milk into a glass or ceramic bowl.
2. Add the sandalwood and ylang-ylang essential oils to the milk, and stir to combine.
3. Add this blend to a warm bath.

SPRAY BLEND

1 ounce distilled water
3 drops lavender essential oil
1 drop clary sage essential oil

1 drop geranium essential oil
1 drop peppermint essential oil

1. Pour the distilled water into a small glass spray bottle.
2. Add the lavender, clary sage, geranium, and peppermint essential oils to the water, and shake well to blend.
3. Spray this blend at home, or use it in an area of your workplace where your coworkers won't be exposed to the scent without their knowledge or permission.

Arthritis

An application of essential oils can bring relief to stiff, aching joints whenever and wherever the pain of arthritis strikes.

NUMBING BLEND

1 teaspoon evening primrose carrier oil
10 drops wintergreen or clove essential oil

1. Pour the evening primrose carrier oil into a small glass or ceramic bowl.
2. Add the wintergreen essential oil to the carrier oil, and stir to combine.
3. Using your fingertips, apply this blend to the affected area, and massage it into the skin.

COOLING BLEND

1 teaspoon evening primrose carrier oil
6 drops Douglas fir essential oil
6 drops eucalyptus essential oil

1. Pour the evening primrose carrier oil into a small glass or ceramic bowl.
2. Add the Douglas fir and eucalyptus essential oils to the carrier oil, and stir to combine.
3. Using your fingertips, apply this blend to the affected area, and massage it into the skin.

2 or 3 drops German chamomile, lemon, or tea tree essential oil

Using a cotton ball, apply the undiluted German chamomile essential oil directly to the affected joint.

Asthma

For people with asthma, the struggle to breathe is worse than uncomfortable—it's exhausting and can be quite frightening, whether the person suffering from this condition is a child or an adult. The search for relief has led to the development of rescue inhalers containing beta-agonist drugs, and other medications also play a role in controlling the symptoms of asthma. Essential oils, too, can relax stressed bronchial pathways while calming the anxiety that accompanies the fight for air.

2 tablespoons vegetable carrier oil
5 drops cypress essential oil
5 drops frankincense essential oil
5 drops geranium essential oil

1. Pour the vegetable carrier oil into a small glass or ceramic bowl.
2. Add the cypress, frankincense, and geranium essential oils to the carrier oil, and stir to combine.
3. Use this blend to massage the back, moving your hands with firm but gentle strokes from the base of the spine up to the shoulders and then over the shoulders and down the sides.

3 cups hot water
¼ teaspoon eucalyptus, lavender, or peppermint essential oil

1. Pour the hot water into a glass or ceramic bowl.
2. Add the eucalyptus oil (it will remain on the water's surface).

3. Drape a towel over your head in such a way that it is also draped closely over the bowl.
4. Bend to hold your face over the bowl, and breathe deeply. *Keep your eyes closed.*
5. Remain in this position until the water cools, periodically lifting one side of the towel to take a breath of fresh air.
6. Repeat this treatment as desired, starting with a fresh bowl of hot water and perhaps a different essential oil.

RUB

1 ounce vegetable carrier oil
6 drops lavender essential oil
4 drops geranium essential oil
1 drop marjoram essential oil
1 drop peppermint essential oil

1. Pour the vegetable carrier oil into a small glass or ceramic bowl.
2. Add the lavender, geranium, marjoram, and peppermint essential oils to the carrier oil, and stir to combine.
3. At bedtime, rub this blend on the chest.[3]

Athlete's Foot

Athlete's foot is a fungal infection that can cause the skin of your feet to itch, peel, and flake. You can relieve the symptoms, and you can help the situation by wearing only cotton or wool socks. But the most effective approach is to kill the yeast that causes the infection. With essential oils, you can relieve the symptoms and treat the infection at the same time.

DAB-ON BLEND

1 ounce carrier oil
6 drops tea tree essential oil
3 drops lavender essential oil

1. Pour the carrier oil into a small glass or ceramic bowl.

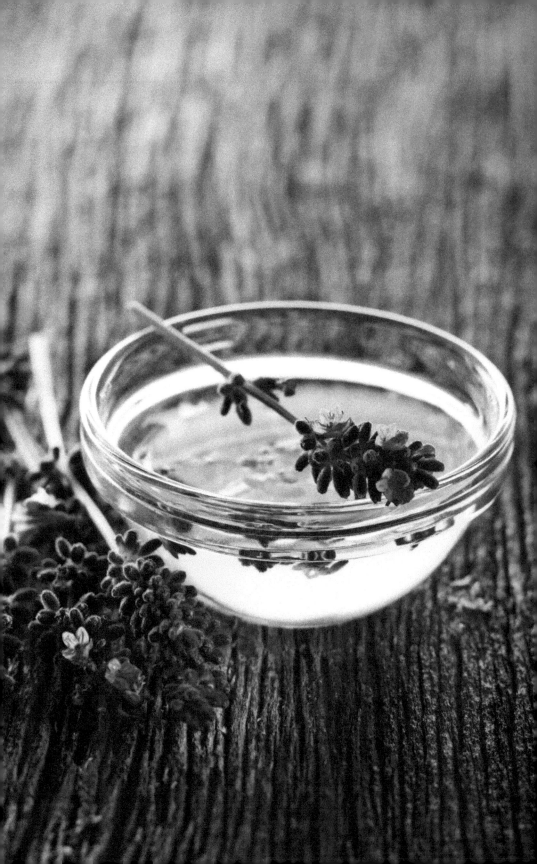

2. Add the tea tree and lavender essential oils to the carrier oil, and stir to combine.
3. Using a cotton swab, dab this blend on the affected areas, especially between the toes, where the infection originates.
4. Put on a clean pair of cotton socks.
5. Repeat this treatment 3 times daily, and continue the treatment for at least 1 week after symptoms disappear.

SOAK

Warm water
1 cup salt
5 drops tea tree essential oil

1. Fill a large glass or ceramic bowl with warm water. The bowl should be large enough to hold both feet.
2. Pour the salt into a glass or ceramic bowl.
3. Add the tea tree essential oil to the salt, and stir to combine.
4. Add the oil mixture to the water, and stir to dissolve.
5. Soak your feet in this mixture for at least 5 minutes.
6. Remove your feet from the water, and dry them thoroughly.
7. Apply the dab-on blend for athlete's foot (page 69).
8. Repeat this treatment daily until symptoms disappear.

POWDER

1 cup dry green clay (available in powdered form at natural foods stores)
10 drops tea tree essential oil

1. Put the clay in the glass jar of a blender that has an opening in the lid.
2. Add the tea tree essential oil 2 drops at a time through the blender's opening, pulsing the blender until all the oil has been added.
3. Turn the blender to the "mix" setting, and allow it to run for 1 minute so the clay and oil are thoroughly combined.
4. Apply this powder once a day to your feet, especially to the spaces between your toes.

Back Pain

Everyone has it, whether from hunching over a keyboard or standing behind a checkout counter and asking whether customers want paper or plastic bags. If you know that the source of your back pain is the normal wear and tear of life, and not a ruptured or herniated disk or a degenerative disease, a combination of massage, rest, and essential oils can get you feeling like your old self again.

RUB

2 tablespoons avocado or olive carrier oil
10 drops marjoram essential oil
10 drops rosemary essential oil
10 drops sage essential oil

1. Pour the avocado carrier oil into a small glass or ceramic bowl.
2. Add the marjoram, rosemary, and sage essential oils to the carrier oil, and stir to combine.
3. Rub (or have someone rub) this blend into the muscles of your back.

NEAT BLEND

10 drops basil essential oil
10 drops cypress essential oil

1. Using a dropper, transfer the basil and cypress essential oils into a small glass or ceramic bowl, and stir to combine.
2. Using your fingers, apply this undiluted blend at least 3 times a day to the affected area.

SOAK

½ cup salt
10 drops clary sage essential oil
10 drops lavender essential oil

1. Pour the salt into a glass or ceramic bowl.

2. Add the clary sage and lavender essential oils to the salt, and stir to combine.
3. Add the mixture to a bathtub filled with warm water, and stir to dissolve.
4. Soak for 15 to 20 minutes.

Bee Sting

At the very least, a sting means discomfort, redness, and localized swelling, especially if the stinger is still in the skin. But a bee sting can also cause pain, fever, headache, and swelling beyond the site of the sting. If you get stung, use a magnifying glass to locate the stinger, and then remove the stinger with a pair of tweezers (in a pinch, use the corner of a credit card). Once the stinger is out, you can apply a cold pack to the sting site or soothe it with an application of an essential oil that has antihistamine and anti-inflammatory properties.

WHEN TO SEE A DOCTOR People who are allergic to bee stings can experience an anaphylactic reaction, which may include such life-threatening symptoms as difficulty breathing, rapid pulse, a sharp drop in blood pressure, shock, and even cardiac arrest. An anaphylactic reaction requires emergency medical treatment.

COLD PACK

1 pint refrigerated water
11 drops chamomile oil

1. Pour the water into a glass or ceramic bowl or low basin.
2. Add 10 drops of chamomile essential oil to the water.
3. Follow the instructions in chapter 3 for making a cold pack (page 46).
4. Keep the cold pack in place over the sting for 3 to 4 hours, replacing the water with freshly refrigerated water as necessary.
5. After 3 to 4 hours, remove the cold pack, and apply 1 drop of chamomile essential oil directly to the site of the sting.

1 drop chamomile essential oil

After treatment with the cold pack, apply 1 drop of undiluted chamomile oil directly to the sting site 3 times a day until the swelling and pain are gone.

NEAT TREATMENT

1 drop lavender, peppermint, or wintergreen essential oil

1. For the first hour after the sting, apply 1 drop of undiluted lavender essential oil every 15 minutes to the site of the sting.
2. After the first hour, apply 1 drop of undiluted lavender essential oil 3 times a day to the site of the sting until discomfort is gone.

Black Toenail

Ballet dancers, soccer players, and place kickers know all about this problem, but someone from a less glamorous walk of life can stub an unprotected big toe and end up with the same type of big black bruise under the nail. If the nail is loose, it should be removed by a podiatrist. A nail that is still intact can be treated with essential oils. (If you're looking for information about treating toenail fungus, see "Toenail Fungus," page 187).

NEAT TREATMENT

1 or 2 drops hyssop essential oil

Using a dropper, apply 1 or 2 drops of undiluted hyssop essential oil as far under the toenail as you can.

TOENAIL BLEND

1 teaspoon carrier oil
5 drops hyssop essential oil

1. Pour the carrier oil into a small glass or ceramic bowl.
2. Add the hyssop essential oil to the carrier oil, and stir to combine.
3. Rub this blend on the affected toe and toenail.

Blisters

Fluid trapped under the skin forms a blister, which is something like a bubble on the skin's surface. Whatever the cause—poorly fitting shoes, athlete's foot, or a virus like herpes simplex—a blister can be quite painful if it eventually breaks, and the delicate new skin underneath can become infected.

NEAT TREATMENT

If the blister has not broken

1 drop lavender or chamomile essential oil

1. Gently clean the affected area with mild soap and warm water.
2. Apply 1 drop of undiluted lavender essential oil to the blister.
3. Cover the blister with a gauze pad, using first aid tape to hold the pad in place.

If the blister has broken

1 or 2 drops German chamomile essential oil

1. Carefully trim away the dead skin once it has lifted on its own from the blistered spot.
2. Apply the undiluted German chamomile essential oil directly to the healing skin once a day until the skin toughens up.

DISINFECTANT BLEND

If the blister has broken

2 drops carrier oil
1 drop lavender essential oil
1 drop tea tree essential oil

1. Pour the carrier oil into a small glass or ceramic bowl.
2. Add the lavender and tea tree essential oils to the carrier oil, and stir to combine.
3. Using a cotton swab, gently dab this blend on the healing skin.
4. Cover the healing skin with an adhesive bandage, or use a doughnut-shaped moleskin to protect the area if the broken blister is on your foot and you need to wear shoes.

Blood Vessels (Broken)

Sometimes called spider veins, these thin red, blue, or purple lines that appear on the face, cheeks, nose, arms, and legs are caused by broken blood vessels. They can be the result of aging, childbirth, sun damage, rosacea, or hormonal changes. They'll heal and fade on their own in three weeks or so, but essential oils can support the healing process.

MOISTURIZING BLEND

4 ounces unscented skin moisturizer or lotion
10 drops Roman chamomile or rose essential oil

1. Pour the moisturizer into a small glass or ceramic bowl.
2. Add the Roman chamomile essential oil to the moisturizer, and stir to combine.
3. Smooth this blend on the affected area 2 or 3 times daily until the broken vessels fade.

COLD PACK

1 pint refrigerated water
10 drops helichrysum, Roman chamomile, or rose essential oil

1. Pour the water into a glass or ceramic bowl or low basin.
2. Add the helichrysum essential oil to the water.
3. Follow the instructions in chapter 3 for making a cold pack (page 46).
4. Remove the cold pack when it warms to body temperature.

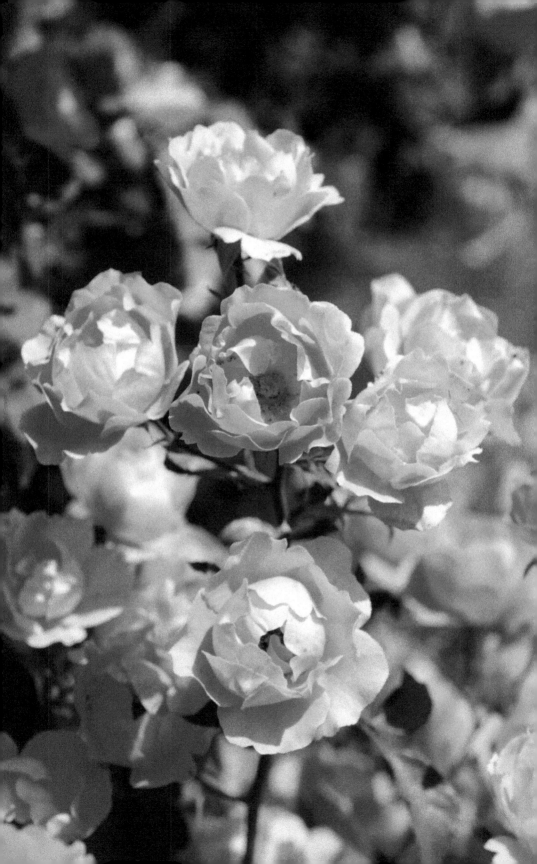

5. Repeat this treatment 2 or 3 times a day until the lines from the broken blood vessels have faded.

MASSAGE BLEND

1 ounce olive, sunflower, or sweet almond carrier oil
25 drops cypress essential oil

1. Pour the olive carrier oil into a small glass or ceramic bowl.
2. Add the cypress essential oil to the carrier oil, and stir to combine.
3. Using your fingertips, apply this blend to the area above the broken blood vessel, and massage into the skin. (Avoid massaging below the blood vessel—that puts more pressure on the capillary and can prolong the healing process.)
4. Repeat this treatment 2 or 3 times a day until the lines from the broken blood vessels have faded.

Body Odor

Bacteria just love sweaty skin, and body odor is the natural consequence. The chemicals in commercial deodorant sprays and sticks can be effective against body odor, but essential oils offer a more natural alternative.

SPRAY DEODORANT

3 ounces grain alcohol (Everclear is recommended)
30 drops essential oil (good choices: lavender, lemon, peppermint, or tea tree)

1. Pour the grain alcohol into a 3-ounce glass spray bottle.
2. Add the essential oil to the alcohol, and shake well.
3. Spray this deodorant under your arms after a shower.[4]

DEODORANT STICK

See the recipe in chapter 5 for making your own deodorant stick with essential oils (page 204).

Boils

An ingrown hair, a clogged sweat gland, a splinter, or another type of lesion can erupt into a boil, an infection (usually staphylococcus) on the surface of the skin that often turns into a nasty, painful lump. Left untreated, the boil can become even more painful, and the infection can spread. Treatment with essential oils that have antibiotic properties can help nip a boil in the bud.

NEAT TREATMENT

If the boil is small and has not become inflamed

2 drops lavender essential oil

1. Using a cotton ball, apply the undiluted lavender essential oil directly to the boil 3 times a day.
2. Repeat this treatment until the boil disappears.

NEAT BLEND

If the boil has erupted and contains pus

5 drops frankincense essential oil
5 drops geranium essential oil
5 drops helichrysum essential oil

1. Transfer the frankincense, geranium, and helichrysum essential oils into a small glass or ceramic bowl, and stir to combine.
2. Using a cotton ball, apply this undiluted blend to the boil.
3. Repeat this treatment 3 times a day until the boil disappears.

Bruises

A bruise appears when capillaries break just under the skin, often after forceful contact between a body part (such as the shin) and an object (such as a table). For the most part, bruises are minor wounds that heal and fade on their own over time, but you can use essential oils in a cold pack to stop a new bruise from spreading, and you can promote fading and circulation by using essential oils in ointments and massage blends.

COLD PACK FOR A BRAND-NEW BRUISE

1 pint cold water
3 drops marjoram essential oil
3 drops Roman chamomile essential oil

1. Pour the water into a glass or ceramic bowl or low basin.
2. Add the Roman chamomile and marjoram essential oils to the water.
3. Follow the instructions in chapter 3 for making a cold pack (page 46).
4. Apply the cold pack within the first hour of bruising.

OINTMENT

2 tablespoons unscented carrier cream
2 drops of calendula essential oil
3 drops lavender essential oil
2 drops helichrysum essential oil
2 drops Roman chamomile essential oil

1. Put the carrier cream in a small glass or ceramic bowl.
2. Add the calendula essential oil, followed by the lavender, helichrysum, and Roman chamomile essential oils, and stir to combine.
3. Using your fingertips, apply this ointment to the bruise 2 or 3 times a day until the bruise fades.[5]

MASSAGE BLEND

1 teaspoon carrier oil
3 drops rosemary essential oil

1. Pour the carrier oil into a small glass or ceramic bowl.
2. Add the rosemary essential oil, and stir to combine.
3. Using your fingertips, apply this blend to the bruise, gently massaging outward from the bruise's center.[6]

Bunions

A bunion occurs when the fluid-filled sac on the first joint of the big toe becomes inflamed and causes the joint to enlarge and protrude. Some women develop bunions from wearing high-heeled shoes, but genetic factors also appear to play a role. A bunion is a nuisance at best, since finding shoes that will accommodate a bunion can be difficult, and at worst a bunion can become swollen and painful. Essential oils won't remove a bunion, but they can soothe the inflammation and help reduce swelling.

NEAT TREATMENT

3 or 4 drops essential oil (good choices: balsam fir, frankincense, lavender, lemon, Roman chamomile, spruce, or wintergreen)

1. Using your fingertips, apply the undiluted essential oil directly to the affected area, gently massaging the oil into the bunion.
2. Cover the bunion with a warm, moist washcloth.
3. Remove the washcloth when it cools to body temperature.
4. Repeat this procedure 2 or 3 times a day, especially upon awakening and at bedtime.[7]

ANTI-INFLAMMATORY BLEND

1 teaspoon vegetable carrier oil
6 drops eucalyptus essential oil
4 drops raven essential oil
3 drops lemon essential oil
1 drop wintergreen essential oil

1. Pour the vegetable carrier oil into a dark-colored glass bottle that closes tightly.
2. Add the eucalyptus, raven, lemon, and wintergreen essential oils to the carrier oil, and stir to combine.
3. Apply 2 drops to the bunion 2 or 3 times a day until the inflammation is relieved.

Warm water
½ cup Epsom salt
2 drops lemon essential oil

1. Pour enough warm water to cover your ankles into a glass or ceramic bowl or basin.
2. Add the Epsom salt to the water.
3. Put your feet in the water, and soak for 20 minutes.
4. Remove your feet from the water, and dry them.
5. Using your fingertips, apply the undiluted lemon essential oil directly to the bunion, and massage gently.

Calluses

A callus is a hardened lump formed by dead cells on the surface of the skin. Rarely painful, a callus forms as a protective layer after repeated contact between the skin (for example, on the sole of the foot) and something hard (such as pebbles on a beach). Calluses appear not only on the feet but also on the hands and even the fingers (guitarists know all about finger calluses). Protective though calluses are, they can become rough, and they can snag or tear socks and stockings. They can even create areas of numbness. Here are some natural remedies to help you reduce or eliminate calluses.

RUB
......

1 teaspoon olive carrier oil
10 drops tea tree essential oil

1. Pour the olive carrier oil into a small glass or ceramic bowl.
2. Add the tea tree essential oil to the carrier oil, and stir to combine.
3. Using a cotton ball, rub this blend into your callus.
4. Repeat this treatment 3 times a day until the callus becomes soft enough to be easily lifted away with a pair of tweezers.

BURNS AND ESSENTIAL OILS
Apply with Caution

The anti-inflammatory and pain-relieving properties found in some essential oils, such as lavender, can help treat first- and second-degree burns, combat infection, and prevent scarring. However, when it comes to third-degree burns, keep essential oils away and leave the treatment of the burns to the professionals. When in doubt, always seek medical attention first.

First-degree burns affect the outer layer of the skin (the epidermis) and are characterized by redness and some pain. Sunburn and minor burns from touching hot appliances fall into this category.

Second-degree burns affect the second layer of the skin (the dermis) and are characterized by broken skin and blisters.

Third-degree burns involve significant tissue damage and demand immediate medical attention to prevent infection and minimize shock. They also call for assessment to determine the requirements for long-term treatment. *Never apply essential oils to a third-degree burn.*

Warm water
5 drops tea tree essential oil

1. Pour enough warm water to cover your ankles into a glass or ceramic bowl or basin.
2. Add the tea tree essential oil to the water.
3. Put your feet in the water, and soak for 10 to 15 minutes, or until the water cools to body temperature.
4. Remove your feet from the water, and dry them.
5. Repeat this treatment until the callus becomes soft enough to be easily lifted away with a pair of tweezers.

OVERNIGHT TREATMENT
....

3 drops tea tree essential oil
1 teaspoon pure aloe vera gel
½ teaspoon turmeric powder

1. Using a cotton ball, rub the callus with the tea tree essential oil.
2. Mix the aloe vera gel with the turmeric powder in a small glass or ceramic bowl.
3. Using your fingertips, apply the mixture to the callus.
4. Cover the callus with a gauze pad, using first aid tape to hold the pad in place, and leave the pad on overnight.
5. Repeat this treatment until the callus becomes soft enough to be easily lifted away with a pair of tweezers.

Cancer

Essential oils cannot cure cancer, and the evidence is poor for essential oils' ability to relieve pain and other symptoms in people who have cancer, although a study published in 2011 does suggest that massage with bitter orange, black pepper, marjoram, patchouli, or rosemary essential oils may help relieve constipation in people with advanced cancer.[8]

Cellulite

The epidermis (outer layer) of a woman's skin is thinner than the outer layer of a man's, and women also tend to have more body fat than most men do. That's why a woman is more likely than a man to have visible cellulite, the lumpy "cottage cheese" skin that results from enlargement of the fat packets just under the epidermis. There's no surefire way to get rid of cellulite, but you can enlist essential oils in breaking down some of that under-the-skin (subcutaneous) fat.

MASSAGE BLEND

1 cup carrier oil
20 drops fennel essential oil
20 drops juniper berry essential oil
10 drops essential oil (good choices: cypress, grapefruit, lemon, rosemary, or sage)

To make the blend

1. Pour the carrier oil into a glass or ceramic bowl.
2. Add the fennel and juniper berry essential oils along with a third essential oil of your choice, and stir to combine.
3. Pour the blend into a dark-colored glass bottle that closes tightly, and store the bottle in the refrigerator between uses.

To use the blend

1. Using your fingertips, apply this blend to areas affected by cellulite, and massage it into the skin.
2. Repeat this treatment once a day for 10 minutes.

Chafing

A sweater, an undergarment, the strap of a shoulder bag, the grip of a golf club—any number of things can rub up against bare skin and cause redness, irritation, and soreness. When a hot spot needs cooling, essential oils can help.

DAB-ON BLEND

1 teaspoon carrier oil
3 or 4 drops helichrysum essential oil

1. Pour the carrier oil into a small glass or ceramic bowl.
2. Add the helichrysum essential oil to the carrier oil, and stir to combine.
3. Using your fingertips, dab this blend on chafed skin and gently rub the blend in, taking care not to further irritate the inflamed area.
4. Repeat this treatment 2 times a day until the skin is back to normal.

NEAT TREATMENT

3 drops tea tree essential oil

1. Moisten a cotton ball with cool water.
2. Using a dropper, apply the undiluted tea tree essential oil to the moistened cotton ball.
3. Press the cotton ball against chafed skin.
4. Repeat this treatment 3 or 4 times a day until the skin is back to normal.

BATH BLEND

2 cups baking soda
10 drops lavender essential oil

1. Run a lukewarm bath.
2. Add the baking soda and the lavender essential oil to the bathwater.
3. Soak for 20 minutes.
4. Repeat this treatment once a day until the skin is back to normal.

Chapped Lips

Cold winds, dry weather, and the heat of summer all take a toll on the lips, as do dehydration and other medical issues. Petroleum-based commercial lip balms may help relieve the cracking and peeling that accompany chapped lips, but those products don't do anything to moisturize lips or prevent further chapping. Here are a few natural remedies that give chapped lips something more than a coat of wax.

SOOTHING ALOE BLEND

1 dab aloe vera gel
1 drop essential oil (good choices: frankincense, lavender, or myrrh)

1. Dispense the aloe vera gel onto your fingertip.
2. Add the essential oil to the aloe vera gel, and smooth the mixture between your finger and your thumb to combine.
3. Using your fingertip, apply this blend to chapped lips as often as desired.

SOOTHING SHEA BUTTER BLEND

1 dab shea butter
1 drop essential oil (good choices: frankincense, lavender, myrrh, or rose hip)

1. Dispense the shea butter onto your fingertip.
2. Add the essential oil to the shea butter, and smooth the mixture between your finger and your thumb to combine.
3. Using your fingertip, apply this blend to chapped lips as often as desired.

LIP BALM

See the recipe in chapter 5 for making your own lip balm with essential oils (page 206).

Chicken Pox

Chicken pox is a viral infection most commonly seen in children that is caused by the same organism responsible for giving shingles to adults. The infection, from start to finish, lasts for about two weeks. The worst part—a fever along with itchy, blistering sores all over the body—goes on for just a few days, but those days can feel like forever to a suffering child. You can use essential oils to soothe your child's skin and make those days less miserable.

BATH BLEND

1 handful oats
3 drops essential oil (good choices: lavender, melissa, peppermint, Roman chamomile, or tea tree)

1. Put the oats inside a small cloth drawstring bag.
2. Add the essential oil to the bag and draw the strings closed.
3. While running a warm bath, place the bag under the tap.
4. Invite your child to soak as long as desired.

ANTI-ITCH CREAM

1 tablespoon witch hazel
2 teaspoons bentonite clay
1 teaspoon fine sea salt
1 teaspoon baking soda
5 drops lavender essential oil
5 drops Melrose blend (from Young Living Essential Oils)
5 drops peppermint essential oil
3 drops Ravensara blend (from Young Living Essential Oils)

1. Put the witch hazel, clay, sea salt, and baking soda in a small glass or ceramic bowl.
2. Add the lavender essential oil, Melrose blend, peppermint essential oil, and Ravensara blend to the bowl, and stir to combine.

3. Using a cotton ball, dab the cream very gently on inflamed pox, taking care not to rub—that could tear off a scab and leave a scar.
4. Repeat this treatment as needed to relieve itching.[9]

1 ounce coconut carrier oil
10 drops helichrysum essential oil
8 drops lemongrass essential oil
6 drops lavender essential oil
5 drops myrrh essential oil
4 drops patchouli essential oil

1. Pour the coconut carrier oil into a small glass or ceramic bowl.
2. Add the helichrysum, lemongrass, lavender, myrrh, and patchouli essential oils to the carrier oil, and stir to combine.
3. Using a cotton ball, dab this blend very gently on the healing skin, taking care not to rub.
4. Repeat this treatment once a day.[10]

Chicken Skin

Keratosis pilaris, the scientific name of this harmless but often distressing condition, is caused by a buildup of a naturally occurring protein (keratin) in the hair follicles and is characterized by persistent tiny red bumps on the arms, legs, and head. There's no cure, and dermatological treatment—cosmetic only, so it's probably not covered by health insurance—involves lasers and lots of money. If you want to keep chicken skin in check without investing in a *Star Wars* arsenal, try these remedies.

PREWASH

1 teaspoon apple cider vinegar

1. Pour the apple cider vinegar onto a wet washcloth.
2. Using the washcloth, moisten your skin before using the exfoliating/moisturizing blend described in this section.

2 tablespoons brown sugar

2 tablespoons granulated sugar

1 tablespoon raw honey

4 tablespoons coconut carrier oil

2 drops lemon essential oil[11]

1. Pour the brown sugar, granulated sugar, and honey into a small glass or ceramic bowl.
2. Add the coconut carrier oil and lemon essential oil to the mixture, and stir to combine.
3. In the shower, scrub vigorously with this blend, using a washcloth, a bath sponge, or a soft loofah to exfoliate your skin.
4. Leave the blend on for 5 minutes to moisturize your skin, then rinse the blend off.

Colds

The common cold is caused by so many different viruses that medical science can't find a broad-spectrum cure for it. But you can prepare for your next cold by stocking up on antiviral and symptom-fighting essential oils like clove, eucalyptus, ginger, lavender, lemon, peppermint, rosemary, tea tree, and thyme.

NEAT INHALER BLEND

1 drop clove essential oil

1 drop eucalyptus essential oil

1 drop peppermint essential oil

1 drop thyme essential oil

1. Add the clove, eucalyptus, peppermint, and thyme essential oils to the wick inside the inhaler.
2. Hold the inhaler up to your nose, and breathe in deeply as often as necessary to keep your nasal passages open.

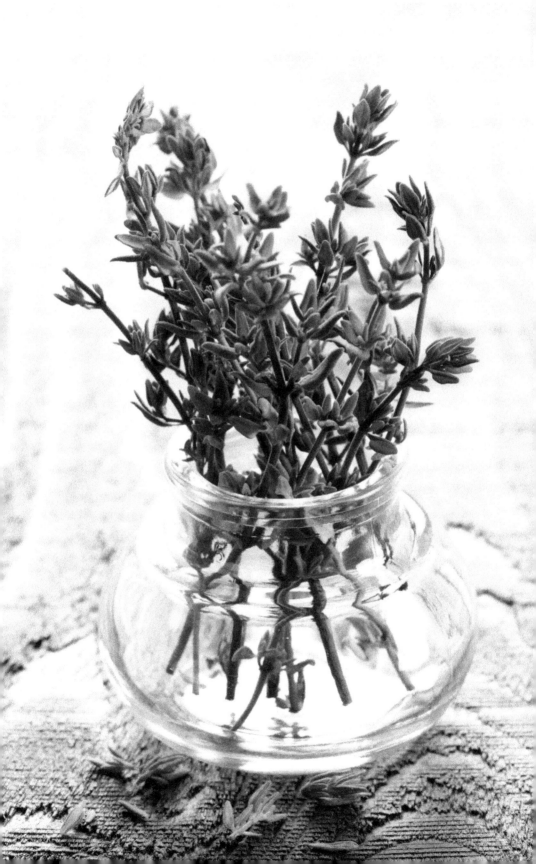

3 cups hot water
1 drop clove essential oil
1 drop lavender essential oil
1 drop tea tree essential oil
1 drop thyme essential oil

1. Pour the hot water into a glass or ceramic bowl.
2. Add the clove, lavender, tea tree, and thyme essential oils (they will remain on the water's surface).
3. Drape a towel over your head in such a way that it is also draped closely over the bowl.
4. Bend to hold your face over the bowl, and breathe deeply. *Keep your eyes closed.*
5. Remain in this position until the water cools, periodically lifting one side of the towel to take a breath of fresh air.
6. Repeat this treatment as desired, starting with a fresh bowl of hot water.

MASSAGE BLEND
·····························

1 teaspoon carrier oil
3 drops rosemary essential oil
2 drops eucalyptus essential oil
1 drop lemon essential oil

1. Pour the carrier oil into a small glass or ceramic bowl.
2. Add the rosemary, eucalyptus, and lemon essential oils to the carrier oil, and stir to combine.
3. Using your fingertips, gently rub this blend on your chest, neck, and cheekbones. You can also rub it around your nose, following the line of your sinus cavities.
4. Repeat this treatment 2 or 3 times a day until symptoms subside.[12]

Cold Sores

The viruses that cause colds and other illnesses can also create cold sores, a form of herpes that can be as painful as it is embarrassing, since cold sores and fever blisters tend to appear on the face, near the lips. Over-the-counter medications have their place, but you can also use natural remedies to promote healing and keep the skin around the sore from cracking.

HEALING BLEND

1 teaspoon grape seed carrier oil
4 drops geranium essential oil
4 drops tea tree essential oil

1. Pour the grape seed carrier oil into a small glass or ceramic bowl.
2. Add the geranium and tea tree essential oils to the carrier oil, and stir to combine.
3. Using a cotton swab, apply this blend to the cold sore.
4. Repeat this treatment 3 or 4 times a day until the sore heals.

SOFTENER

1 teaspoon sunflower carrier oil
2 drops eucalyptus essential oil
2 drops geranium essential oil
2 drops Roman chamomile essential oil

1. Pour the sunflower carrier oil into a small glass or ceramic bowl.
2. Add the eucalyptus, geranium, and Roman chamomile essential oils to the carrier oil, and stir to combine.
3. Using a cotton ball or cotton swab, dab this blend around the cold sore to prevent the affected lip from cracking and to keep the surrounding skin soft.

PAIN-RELIEVING BLEND

1 teaspoon sunflower carrier oil
3 or 4 drops lavender essential oil

1. Pour the sunflower carrier oil into a small glass or ceramic bowl.
2. Add the lavender essential oil to the carrier oil, and stir to combine.
3. Using a cotton ball or cotton swab, dab this blend on the cold sore.
4. Repeat this treatment as necessary to relieve pain.[13]

Colic

When your baby cries uncontrollably for hours at a time and continues to cry this way more than three days a week for several weeks in a row, the likely culprit is colic. Your baby will grow out of it, but here are some remedies to use until that happy day arrives.

MASSAGE BLEND

1 teaspoon sweet almond carrier oil
1 drop geranium or lavender essential oil

1. Pour the sweet almond carrier oil into a small glass or ceramic bowl.
2. Add the geranium essential oil to the carrier oil, and stir to combine.
3. Warm the combined oils in the palm of your hand.
4. Using your fingertips and a circular motion, gently rub this blend over your baby's stomach.
5. When the baby becomes quieter, turn him over on his stomach, and continue the gentle massage on his back. For the same calming effect, you can also rub this blend on your baby's feet.

WARM COMPRESS

1 pint warm water
1 drop geranium or lavender essential oil

1. Follow the instructions in chapter 3 for making a warm compress (page 48).

2. Place the warm compress on your baby's stomach as she lies on her back.
3. Remove the compress when it cools to body temperature.
4. Repeat this treatment if the crying begins again.

Colitis and Crohn's Disease

Colitis and Crohn's disease are chronic autoimmune conditions characterized by inflammation of the colon. Cramping, diarrhea, vomiting, and resulting nutritional deficiencies are all symptoms of both illnesses. Anyone affected by either one needs to be under competent medical care, since they can eventually involve even more serious conditions. Essential oils cannot cure either colitis or Crohn's, but they can help with the symptoms.

BATH BLEND

3 drops basil essential oil (other good choices: marjoram, peppermint, and rosemary)

1. Run a warm bath.
2. Add the basil essential oil to the bathwater. (You can also add the same amount of marjoram, peppermint, or rosemary essential oil, singly or in combination.)
3. Soak until the water cools to body temperature.

MASSAGE BLEND

5 milliliters jojoba carrier oil
3 drops basil essential oil
3 drops marjoram essential oil
3 drops peppermint essential oil

1. Pour the jojoba carrier oil into a small glass or ceramic bowl.
2. Add the basil, marjoram, and peppermint essential oils to the carrier oil, and stir to combine.
3. Using your fingertips, rub this blend over your abdomen to promote bowel function and relieve cramping.

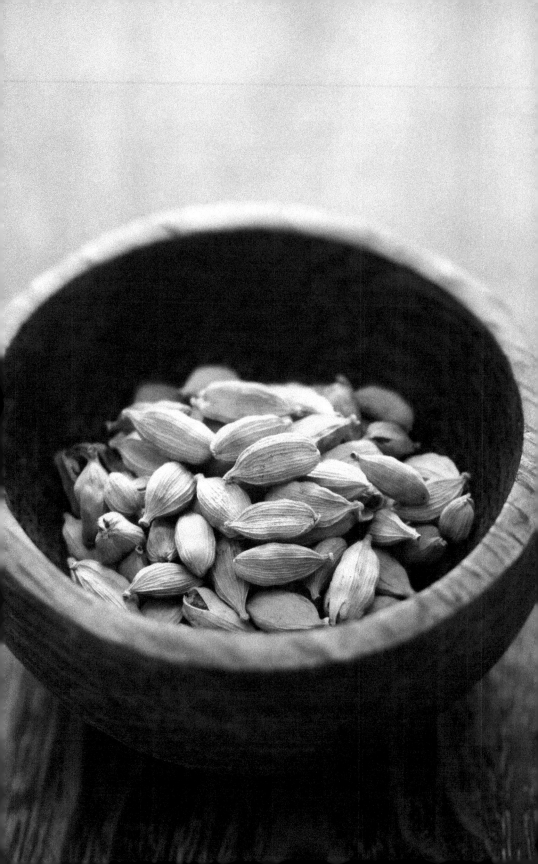

3 drops eucalyptus essential oil

2 drops Roman chamomile essential oil

2 drops neroli essential oil

2 drops peppermint essential oil

1. Add the eucalyptus, chamomile, neroli, and peppermint essential oils to the water in your diffuser.
2. Turn the diffuser on, and let it run for 15 minutes of every hour for as many hours as needed until your system returns to normal.

Constipation

Everyone is different when it comes to what constitutes a normal elimination schedule. But if several days have gone by, constipation may have set in. Here are some natural remedies for getting your system back on track.

MASSAGE BLEND

2 tablespoons carrier oil

15 drops patchouli essential oil

5 drops black pepper essential oil

5 drops cardamom essential oil

1. Pour the carrier oil into a small glass or ceramic bowl.
2. Add the patchouli, black pepper, and cardamom essential oils to the carrier oil, and stir to combine.
3. Using your fingertips and a clockwise circular motion, firmly (but not painfully) massage this blend into your abdomen.
4. Repeat this treatment 3 times a day until your system returns to normal.[14]

BATH BLEND

5 drops lavender essential oil

5 drops rosemary essential oil

1. Run a warm bath.
2. Add the lavender and rosemary essential oils to the bathwater.
3. Soak until the water cools to body temperature.

Corns

Unlike a callus, which is large and flat, a corn is small and often thick, forming a circular shape or a cone that can become irritated and painful. Between toes, corns can be soft and flaky. Whichever kind of corn you have, you're probably eager to get rid of it—and there are simple ways to do that without seeing a podiatrist.

RUB

2 tablespoons carrier oil
10 drops calendula essential oil or 30 drops tagetes essential oil

1. Pour the carrier oil into a small glass or ceramic bowl.
2. Add the calendula essential oil to the carrier oil, and stir to combine.
3. Using your fingertips, rub this blend gently over the corn.
4. Repeat this treatment 3 times a day for 3 or 4 days until the corn softens.
5. When the corn has softened, slough it away with a foot file or a pumice stone.

SOAK

½ cup salt
2 teaspoons apple cider vinegar
5 drops carrot seed essential oil
5 drops tagetes essential oil

1. Pour enough warm water to cover your ankles into a glass or ceramic bowl or basin.
2. Add the salt and apple cider vinegar to the water, and stir to combine.
3. Put your feet in the water, and soak for 20 minutes.

4. Remove your feet from the water, and dry them.
5. Pour the carrot seed and tagetes essential oils into a small glass or ceramic bowl, and stir to combine.
6. Using a cotton ball or a cotton swab, apply 2 drops of this blend to the corn.
7. Repeat this treatment once a day for 3 days until the corn softens.
8. When the corn has softened, slough it away with a foot file or a pumice stone.

Cough

Essential oils can boost the effectiveness of your tried-and-true cough remedies and even give you some new ones.

RUB

1 teaspoon carrier oil
3 drops eucalyptus essential oil
2 drops thyme essential oil

1. Pour the carrier oil into a small glass or ceramic bowl.
2. Add the eucalyptus and thyme essential oils to the carrier oil, and stir to combine.
3. Rub this blend over your chest and back.
4. Repeat this treatment as often as desired.

VAPORIZER TREATMENT

3 drops chamomile essential oil (other choices: frankincense, ginger, lavender, oregano, sandalwood, or tea tree)

1. Add the chamomile essential oil to the water in your vaporizer. (You can also add the same amount of frankincense, ginger, lavender, oregano, sandalwood, or tea tree essential oil, singly or in combination.)
2. Turn the vaporizer on, and let it run for 15 minutes of every hour for as many hours as needed.

Cracked Heels

When winter dries out the air, or when summer scorches an already dry environment, you may find yourself with chapped heels that develop painful cracks. A salve made with essential oils can help heal the cracks while soothing and softening your feet.

EXFOLIATING BLEND

1 cup cornmeal
1 cup dry oatmeal
¼ cup coarse salt
1 teaspoon peppermint essential oil

1. Put the cornmeal, oatmeal, and salt in a small glass or ceramic bowl.
2. Add the peppermint essential oil to the mixture, and stir to combine.
3. Using your fingertips, apply this blend into your heels and the soles of your feet, and massage it into the skin to exfoliate and start the smoothing process.
4. Repeat the treatment once a day until symptoms subside. For best results, rinse the blend off the heels, dry them, and use a pumice stone to smooth any remaining roughness.

SOAK

3 drops lavender essential oil
3 drops lemon essential oil
3 drops rosemary essential oil

1. Pour enough warm water to cover your ankles into a glass or ceramic bowl or basin.
2. Add the lavender, lemon, and rosemary essential oils to the water.
3. Soak for 15 minutes.
4. Repeat this treatment once a day until symptoms subside.[15]

1 tablespoon carrier oil
3 drops lavender essential oil

1. Pour the carrier oil into a small glass or ceramic bowl.
2. Add the lavender essential oil to the carrier oil, and stir to combine.
3. At bedtime, massage this blend into your heels.
4. Put on a pair of cotton socks, and wear them overnight.
5. Repeat this treatment once a day until symptoms subside.

Croup

Croup, very common in children, is a viral infection of the upper respiratory system. It inflames the larynx and causes a recognizable, alarming, barking cough. Croup is very contagious in the first few days, and it's often accompanied by a fever, runny nose, and other cold-like symptoms. The most popular and effective natural remedy for croup is to bundle a child up and take her outside to breathe very cold air (in a wintry climate) or (in a warm one) to stay in the kitchen and let her breathe the cold air of the freezer. Essential oils can also offer some relief from bronchial congestion.

STEAM TREATMENT

3 cups hot water
3 drops eucalyptus essential oil
3 drops peppermint essential oil (for children 2 or over)

1. Pour the hot water into a glass or ceramic bowl.
2. Add the eucalyptus and peppermint essential oils (they will remain on the water's surface).
3. Drape a towel over your child's head in such a way that the towel is also draped closely over the bowl.
4. Have your child bend to hold his face over the bowl while breathing. *Make sure the child keeps his eyes closed.*

5. Have the child remain in this position until the water cools, periodically lifting one side of the towel for him to take a breath of fresh air.
6. After 2 to 3 minutes, take the child outside to breathe fresh outdoor air, a change that will "shock" his breathing passages and restore fairly normal breathing for a while.

WARM COMPRESS

2 drops eucalyptus essential oil
2 peppermint essential oil

1. Follow the instructions in chapter 3 for making a warm compress (page 48).
2. Place the warm compress to the chest.
3. Remove the compress when it cools to body temperature.
4. Repeat this treatment 3 times a day until normal breathing is restored.

VAPORIZER TREATMENT

3 drops cinnamon essential oil
3 drops clove essential oil
3 drops thyme essential oil

1. Add the cinnamon, clove, and thyme essential oils to the water in your vaporizer.
2. Turn the vaporizer on, and allow it to run throughout the day or overnight.

Cuts and Scrapes

A number of essential oils have antiseptic and antibacterial properties that make them effective substitutes for commercial first aid creams and topical antibiotics, often without the sting of an alcohol-based disinfectant. Most cuts and scrapes will heal more quickly in the open air, but a wound should be covered if there's any chance that it could pick up dirt, or that the same spot could be reinjured. A drop or two of an essential oil can be applied directly to the cut or scrape before the bandage goes on.

Lukewarm water
3 or 4 drops lavender essential oil (other choices: eucalyptus, lemon, pine, or tea tree)

1. Fill your sink with lukewarm water.
2. Add the lavender essential oil to the water.
3. Using a washcloth, gently clean the cut or scrape.
4. Gently dry the cut or scrape with a soft, clean towel.

NEAT TREATMENT

1 drop lavender essential oil (other choices: eucalyptus or tea tree)

Using a cotton swab, apply the undiluted lavender essential oil directly to the cut or scrape.

Dandruff

There are lots of dandruff shampoos and medicated products that you can buy, but none will solve the problem permanently. Remarkably, however, essential oils and some changes to your hair-care regimen can go quite a long way toward solving the problem.

ESSENTIAL SHAMPOO

8 ounces unscented shampoo (available at natural foods stores)
10 drops lavender essential oil
4 drops tea tree essential oil

1. Pour the shampoo into an 8-ounce dark-colored glass bottle that closes tightly.
2. Add the lavender and tea tree essential oils to the shampoo, and shake well to blend.

3. Apply a quarter-size amount to your hair.
4. Lather, and wait 30 seconds before rinsing.

OVERNIGHT CONDITIONING BLEND

1 ounce spring water (bottled water)
1 tablespoon apple cider vinegar
5 drops carrot essential oil
5 drops eucalyptus essential oil
5 drops thyme essential oil
3 drops sage essential oil

1. Pour the spring water and apple cider vinegar into a dark-colored glass bottle that closes tightly.
2. Add the carrot, eucalyptus, thyme, and sage essential oils to the bottle, and shake well to blend.
3. At bedtime, pour 1 teaspoon of this blend into the palm of your hand, and massage it into your scalp.
4. Leave the blend in overnight.
5. In the morning, wash your hair with the shampoo described earlier in this section.[16]

OVERNIGHT DERMATITIS BLEND

1 teaspoon jojoba carrier oil
4 drops tea tree essential oil

1. At bedtime, pour the jojoba carrier oil into a teaspoon.
2. Add the tea tree essential oil to the carrier oil.
3. Pour this blend into the palm of your hand, and massage it into your scalp.
4. Leave the blend in overnight.
5. In the morning, wash your hair with the shampoo described earlier in this section.
6. Repeat this treatment every night until your scalp stops itching.

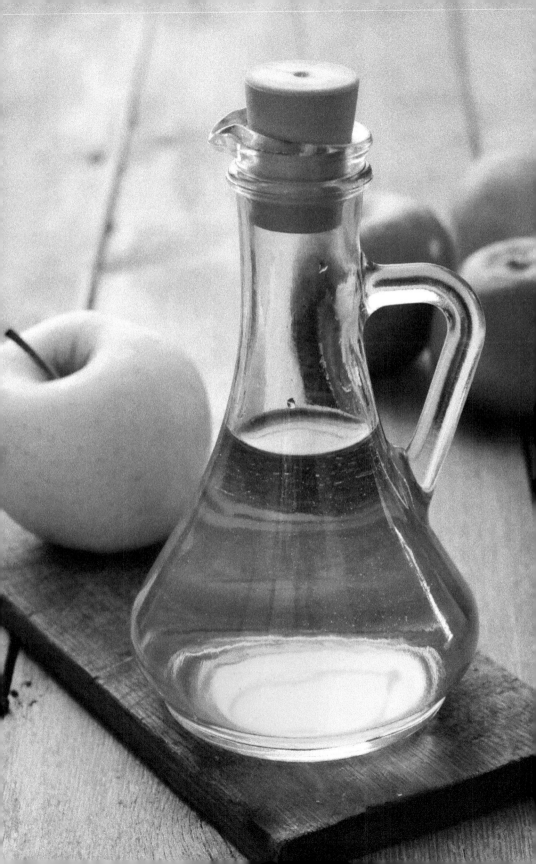

Diabetes

Laboratory research has found that certain essential oils had some positive effects on physiological functions related to insulin production in rats and mice, but these findings have not been tested in clinical trials involving human subjects.[17]

Diaper Rash

Essential oils offer an alternative to using commercial products on a baby's sensitive skin. Here are some remedies that will cool diaper rash and comfort your baby.

CLEANSING BLEND

1 pint warm water
10 drops lavender essential oil
10 drops yarrow essential oil
4 teaspoons jojoba carrier oil

1. Pour the warm water into a glass or ceramic bowl.
2. Transfer the lavender and yarrow essential oils to a dark-colored glass bottle that closes tightly.
3. Add 1 drop of the blended essential oils to the warm water, and stir to blend.
4. Soak a soft cloth in the oil-treated water, and wring out any excess moisture.
5. Using the damp cloth, gently clean the skin affected by diaper rash.
6. Carefully dry the affected skin with a soft, clean towel.
7. Using a cotton ball, smooth a little more of the oil-treated water over the affected skin.
8. Pour the jojoba carrier oil into a second glass or ceramic bowl.
9. Add 1 drop of the blended essential oils to the carrier oil, and stir to combine.

10. Using a cotton ball, apply a light layer of the blended essential and carrier oils to the diaper area.
11. Put a fresh diaper on the baby.

Diarrhea

Someone suffering from diarrhea can lose more than a quart of fluids in a single day, so diarrhea lasting two days or more poses a health risk because of the danger of dehydration. Frequent diarrhea that can't be connected to food poisoning or a virus may indicate a chronic condition that calls for medical intervention. Abdominal massage with essential oils can help resolve ordinary diarrhea.

MASSAGE BLEND

1 teaspoon carrier oil
3 drops lavender essential oil
1 drop eucalyptus essential oil
1 drop tea tree essential oil

1. Pour the carrier oil into a small glass or ceramic bowl.
2. Add the lavender, eucalyptus, and tea tree essential oils to the carrier oil, and stir to combine.
3. Using your fingertips, apply this blend into your abdomen in a circular motion, and massage it into the skin (about 5 minutes).
4. Repeat this treatment 2 times a day.

Dry Skin

The discomforts of dry skin can be easily vanquished with essential oils and carrier oils. The carrier oils moisturize, and the essential oils relieve the itching.

EXFOLIATING SHOWER BLEND

½ cup ground almonds or 1 cup whole almonds
½ cup oatmeal

2 drops evening primrose essential oil
2 drops sandalwood essential oil

1. If you're not starting with ground almonds, put 1 cup of whole almonds in a food processor, and pulse until ground.
2. Transfer the ground almonds to a glass or ceramic bowl.
3. Add the oatmeal along with the evening primrose and sandalwood essential oils to the ground almonds.
4. Transfer the mixture into the glass jar of a blender, and blend to form a paste.
5. Rub this paste vigorously all over your body, paying special attention to dry areas, such as your heels and your elbows.
6. After 1 minute, rinse the paste off in the shower.

MOISTURIZING BATH BLEND

2 tablespoons sweet almond carrier oil
2 teaspoons apricot kernel carrier oil
2 teaspoons avocado carrier oil
50 drops lavender essential oil (other choices: eucalyptus, peppermint, or Roman chamomile)

1. Pour the sweet almond, apricot kernel, and avocado carrier oils into a small glass or ceramic bowl.
2. Add the lavender essential oil to the carrier oils, and stir to combine.
3. Pour the blend into a dark-colored glass bottle that closes tightly.
4. Run a warm bath.
5. Add 1 teaspoon of this blend to the bathwater, and soak as long as you like.[18]

MOISTURIZING SKIN LOTION

1 bottle unscented skin lotion (available at natural foods stores)
10 drops palma rosa essential oil
10 drops rosewood essential oil
5 drops carrot seed essential oil
5 drops German chamomile essential oil

1. Pour the lotion into a dark-colored glass bottle that closes tightly.
2. Add the palma rosa, rosewood, carrot seed, and German chamomile essential oils to the lotion, and shake well.
3. Using your fingertips, apply this blended lotion to your skin.
4. Repeat this treatment 2 times a day until the dryness and itching subside.

Eczema

Eczema, characterized by itchy, inflamed patches on the skin, may arise in response to a new laundry detergent, a scented soap, contact with rough fabrics or with dander from pets, a cold or a case of the flu, prolonged stress, and a variety of other things. Whatever the cause of eczema, its symptoms can be soothed by the right essential oils.

ANTI-INFLAMMATORY BLEND

4 ounces warm water
5 drops chamomile essential oil

1. Pour the water into a small glass or ceramic bowl.
2. Add the chamomile essential oil to the water, and stir to combine.
3. Put a piece of gauze in the water, and let it become saturated.
4. Remove the gauze, and apply it to the affected skin.
5. Leave the gauze in place for 20 minutes.
6. Repeat this treatment as needed until the inflammation subsides.

ANTI-ITCH BLEND

1 tablespoon coconut carrier oil
2 drops frankincense essential oil
2 drops helichrysum essential oil
1 drop geranium essential oil
1 drop thyme essential oil

1. Pour the coconut carrier oil into a small glass or ceramic bowl.
2. Add the frankincense, helichrysum, geranium, and thyme essential oils to the carrier oil, and stir to combine.

3. Using your fingertips, apply this blend to the affected area.
4. Cover the treated area with gauze, or with cotton gloves or socks (if the inflammation is on your hands or feet).
5. Leave the covering on the affected area all day, or reapply the treatment up to 3 times throughout the day.
6. Repeat this treatment as needed until the itching subsides.

OVERNIGHT SOOTHING BLEND

1 tablespoon avocado or jojoba carrier oil
2 drops frankincense essential oil
2 drops helichrysum essential oil
1 drop geranium essential oil
1 drop thyme essential oil

1. Pour the avocado carrier oil into a small glass or ceramic bowl.
2. Add the frankincense, helichrysum, geranium, and thyme essential oils to the carrier oil, and stir to combine.
3. Using your fingertips, apply this blend to the affected area.
4. Cover the treated area with gauze, or with cotton gloves or socks (if the inflammation is on your hands or feet).
5. Repeat the treatment nightly until the inflammation subsides.

Fatigue

The best cure for fatigue is sleep, but that's not always an option. Here's a quick way to keep going when your eyelids have other ideas.

NEAT INHALER BLEND

2 drops ginger essential oil
2 drops lime essential oil

1. Add the undiluted ginger and lime essential oils to the wick inside an inhaler.
2. Hold the inhaler up to your nose, and breathe in deeply as often as necessary to stay refreshed and alert.

Fever

Any fever means not feeling well. You may be dizzy, have no appetite, and be alternately sweating and shivering. Some essential oils can actually help reduce a fever. Others are good at relieving a fever's accompanying symptoms.

RUB

1 teaspoon jojoba carrier oil (or 1 tablespoon for a child)
2 drops lime essential oil (or 1 drop for a child)

1. Pour the jojoba carrier oil into a small glass or ceramic bowl.
2. Add the lime essential oil to the carrier oil, and stir to combine.
3. Using a cotton ball, apply this blend to the soles of the feet.
4. Repeat this treatment every 30 minutes as needed until the fever is reduced.

FEVER-COOLING NEAT TREATMENT

3 or 4 drops peppermint essential oil

1. Using a cotton ball, apply the undiluted peppermint essential oil to the back of the neck or the soles of the feet.
2. Repeat this treatment every 30 minutes as needed until the fever is reduced.

SAFETY REMINDER: CHILDREN AND PEPPERMINT

Peppermint essential oil is not for use with children younger than seven. If you use peppermint oil with older children, never use it undiluted. Instead, dilute half the amount of peppermint oil you would use for an adult in three times the amount of carrier oil that would be appropriate for an adult dose of peppermint oil.

COLD PACK FOR ADULTS AND CHILDREN 3 AND OLDER

1 cup refrigerated water
3 drops lavender essential oil
1 drop eucalyptus essential oil

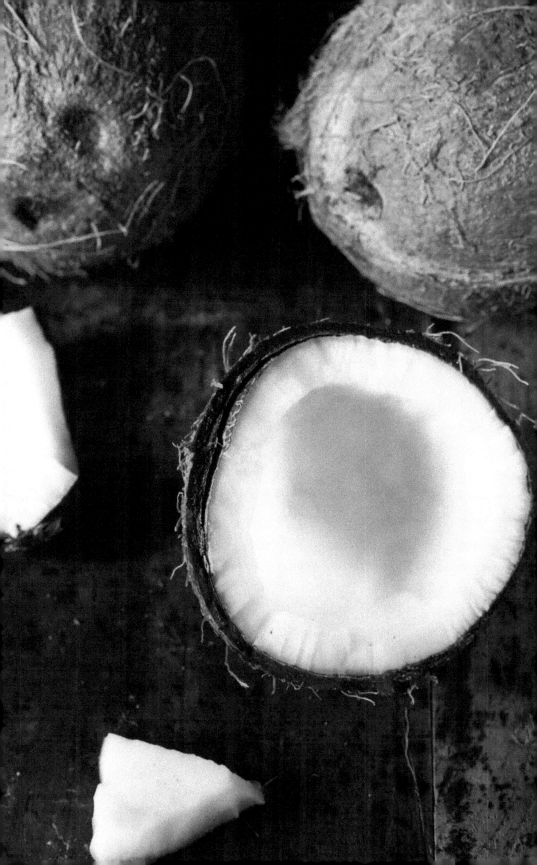

1. Pour the refrigerated water into a glass or ceramic bowl or low basin.
2. Add the lavender and eucalyptus essential oils to the water.
3. Follow the instructions in chapter 3 for making a cold pack (page 46).
4. Place the cold pack on the forehead.
5. Keep the cold pack in place until it warms to body temperature.
6. Repeat this treatment as needed until the fever is reduced.

WHEN TO SEE A DOCTOR A baby younger than eight weeks old who has a fever higher than 100.4 degrees needs to see a pediatrician right away. A doctor should also be consulted if an older child with no other obvious symptoms has a fever that has lasted for two or three days. Any child with a fever that has gone on for more than five days needs to see a doctor.

Fibromyalgia

Fibromyalgia is a chronic, painful condition that affects points throughout the body, including the neck, back, shoulders, pelvis, and hands. The causes of fibromyalgia have not yet been pinpointed, and medications have been only partially effective. Essential oils offer a natural approach to treating the pain, fatigue, and physical and mental stress that accompany this poorly understood condition. If massage is used as a treatment, it's important to seek out a massage therapist who has experience with fibromyalgia, and deep-tissue massages should be avoided.

ANTI-INFLAMMATORY MASSAGE BLEND

1 ounce coconut carrier oil
3 or 4 drops helichrysum essential oil
3 or 4 drops peppermint essential oil
3 or 4 drops spike lavender essential oil

1. Pour the coconut carrier oil into a small glass or ceramic bowl.

2. Add the helichrysum, peppermint, and spike lavender essential oils to the carrier oil, and stir to combine.
3. Using your fingertips, apply this blend to the affected area, and gently massage it into the skin.
4. Repeat this treatment once a day to relieve inflammation.[19]

BROAD-SPECTRUM-RELIEF MASSAGE BLEND

1 ounce carrier oil
4 drops lavender essential oil
4 drops sweet orange essential oil
1 drop frankincense essential oil
1 drop neroli essential oil

1. Pour the carrier oil into a small glass or ceramic bowl.
2. Add the lavender, sweet orange, frankincense, and neroli essential oils to the carrier oil, and stir to combine.
3. Using your fingertips, apply this blend to the affected area, and gently massage it into the skin.
4. Repeat this treatment once a day.[20]

Flatulence

Flatulence, the condition of having gas in the stomach or intestine, is a daily fact of life for everyone, but it can be accompanied by bloating and cramping. In the apothecary of essential oils, there's no better remedy for flatulence than peppermint oil, which is absorbed into the skin and can help relieve gas and indigestion.

GAS-RELIEVING NEAT TREATMENT

4 to 6 drops peppermint essential oil

1. Place the undiluted peppermint essential oil in the palm of one hand.
2. Rub your hands together, and then rub both palms over the skin of your stomach and the area around your navel.
3. Repeat this treatment as often as necessary.

Flu

Even though influenza viruses are highly contagious, you can take protective measures, from conscientiously washing your hands to getting an annual vaccination. But sometimes you get the flu anyway. That's when essential oils can help you weather the storm, especially when you use them in a humidifier, since flu viruses thrive in a cool, dry environment.

HUMIDIFIER TREATMENT

5 drops essential oil (good choices: cinnamon, eucalyptus, frankincense, lavender, lemon, melissa, oregano, peppermint, ravensara, rosemary, sage, tea tree, or thyme)

1. Add one or a blend of the essential oils to the water in your humidifier.
2. Turn the humidifier on, and let it run all day and overnight.
3. Clean the humidifier and repeat this treatment for 3 to 5 days, or until the congestion is relieved.

NEAT PREVENTIVE SHOWER BLEND

10 drops eucalyptus essential oil
10 drops oregano essential oil
10 drops peppermint essential

1. Using a dropper, put the undiluted eucalyptus, oregano, and peppermint essential oils on a wet washcloth.
2. Put the washcloth on the floor of your shower.
3. Turn the water on, and stay in the shower for 15 minutes, breathing deeply.[21]

Foot Odor

When your feet smell, even you don't feel like walking a mile in your own shoes. Keeping your feet clean and dry goes a long way toward controlling foot odor, but if you want to go the extra mile, try these fast-acting remedies.

ANTIBACTERIAL BLEND

1 teaspoon carrier oil
5 drops tea tree essential oil

1. Pour the carrier oil into a small glass or ceramic bowl.
2. Add the tea tree essential oil to the carrier oil, and stir to combine.
3. Using a cotton ball, apply this blend to your feet, taking care to swab between your toes.
4. Repeat this treatment 2 times a day until foot odor is under control.

ANTIBACTERIAL SHOE POWDER

3 tablespoons baking soda
4 drops tea tree essential oil

1. Put the baking soda in a dark-colored glass jar that closes tightly.
2. Add the tea tree essential oil to the baking soda 1 drop at a time to prevent clumping and leave the baking soda as dry as possible.
3. Close the jar tightly, and shake well.
4. Sprinkle ½ teaspoon of the powder into your shoes to absorb moisture, kill bacteria, and destroy any unpleasant odor.
5. Leave the powder in the shoes overnight, then shake it in the morning before wearing.

FRESHENING SHOE SPRAY

4 ounces distilled or spring water
10 drops tea tree essential oil

5 drops geranium essential oil

5 drops sage essential oil

1. Pour the distilled water into a small glass spray bottle.
2. Add the tea tree, geranium, and sage essential oils to the water, and shake well to blend.
3. Use this spray on the insides of your sneakers and other shoes.

Foot Pain

If you're on your feet all day, they tend to hurt by the time evening rolls around. Essential oils can relieve the pain, improve circulation, prevent calluses, and get your feet in shape for the day to come.

SOAK

Warm water

3 drops German chamomile essential oil

3 drops lavender essential oil

3 drops peppermint essential oil

1. Pour enough warm water to cover your ankles into a glass or ceramic bowl or basin.
2. Add the chamomile, lavender, and peppermint essential oils to the water.
3. Put your feet in the water, and soak for 10 to 15 minutes.
4. Remove your feet from the water, and dry them thoroughly.
5. Repeat this treatment once a day, in the evening.

AFTER-SOAK LOTION

½ cup sweet almond carrier oil

¼ cup coconut carrier oil

¼ cup beeswax

1 teaspoon vitamin E oil

2 tablespoons cocoa butter

20 drops eucalyptus essential oil

20 drops peppermint essential oil

To make the lotion

1. Pour the sweet almond and coconut carrier oils into a 1-pint Mason jar.
2. Add the beeswax, vitamin E oil, cocoa butter, and eucalyptus and peppermint essential oils.
3. Fill a saucepan with several inches of water, and place the saucepan over medium heat.
4. Loosely put the lid on the jar, and place the jar in the pan of heating water to melt the lotion ingredients.
5. As the water heats, stir the ingredients to combine them.
6. When all the ingredients have melted and are fully combined, remove the jar from the heat and let the lotion cool.
7. Pour the cooled lotion into a dark-colored glass jar that closes tightly, and store it in the refrigerator between uses.
8. For best results, use within 6 months.

To use the lotion

1. Remove the lotion from the refrigerator and allow it to come to room temperature.
2. After your evening foot soak, dry your feet thoroughly.
3. Using your fingertips, apply a small amount of lotion into your feet, and massage it into your skin.
4. Repeat this treatment once a day, in the evening.[22]

Freckles

Freckles come from a combination of genetics and exposure to the sun. You can't do anything about your genetic profile, but you can wear a good sunscreen to keep freckles to a minimum, and you can use essential oils to fade the freckles you can't avoid, although it may take a few weeks for you to see results.

¼ cup coconut carrier oil

6 drops frankincense essential oil

6 drops lavender essential oil

6 drops myrrh essential oil

To make the blend

1. Pour the coconut carrier oil into a small glass or ceramic bowl.
2. Add the frankincense, lavender, and myrrh essential oils to the carrier oil, and stir to combine.
3. Pour the blend into a dark-colored glass bottle that closes tightly, and store the bottle in the refrigerator between uses.

To use the blend

1. Remove the blend from the refrigerator and allow it to come to room temperature.
2. Using a cotton ball, apply this blend to skin affected by freckles.
3. Repeat this treatment once a day for several weeks, or until your freckles become less noticeable.

1 ounce castor carrier oil

10 drops frankincense essential oil

To make the blend

1. Pour the castor carrier oil into a small glass or ceramic bowl.
2. Add the frankincense essential oil to the carrier oil, and stir to combine.
3. Pour the blend into a dark-colored glass bottle that closes tightly, and store the bottle in the refrigerator between uses.

To use the blend

1. Using a cotton ball, apply this blend to skin affected by freckles.
2. Repeat this treatment 2 times a day for 4 weeks, or until your freckles become less noticeable.

20 drops avocado carrier oil

6 drops sandalwood essential oil

4 drops blue cypress essential oil

4 drops lavender essential oil

4 drops nutmeg essential oil

To make the blend

1. Pour the avocado carrier oil into a small glass or ceramic bowl.
2. Add the sandalwood, blue cypress, lavender, and nutmeg essential oils to the carrier oil, and stir to combine.
3. Pour the blend into a dark-colored glass bottle that closes tightly, and store the bottle in the refrigerator between uses.

To use the blend

1. Using a cotton ball, apply 2 to 4 drops of this blend to skin affected by freckles.
2. Repeat this treatment 3 times a day for 2 weeks, or until your freckles become less noticeable.

Ganglion Cysts

A ganglion cyst is a common, benign, fluid-filled mass that forms for poorly understood reasons on the hand, usually on the back of the wrist. Ganglion cyst generally don't require treatment and will dissipate on their own over time. But if you have one that hurts, interferes with your daily routine, or is just plain unattractive, try treating it with essential oils.

NEAT TREATMENT

2 drops frankincense essential oil

1. Apply the undiluted frankincense essential oil directly to a cyst that is visibly close to the surface.
2. Repeat this treatment 2 or 3 times a day until the cyst disappears.

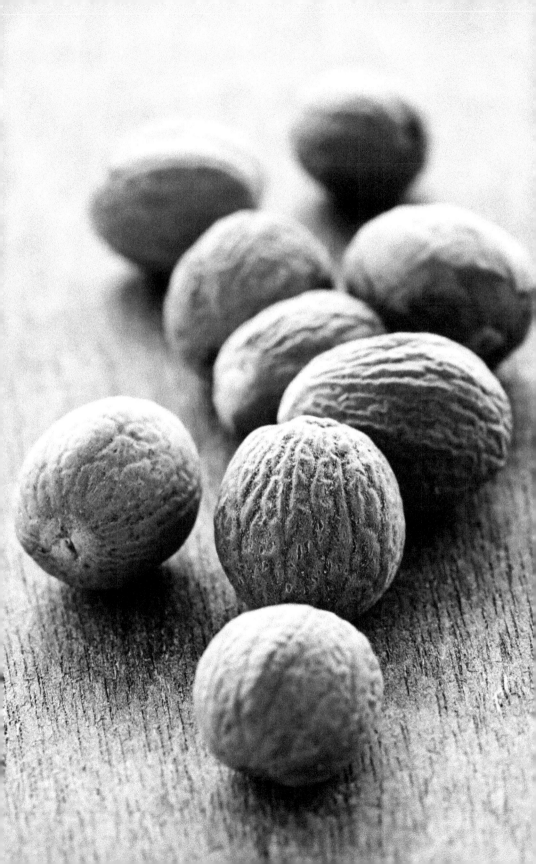

Gout

This painful inflammation is caused by a buildup of uric acid crystals in a single joint, most often in a hand or a foot. Gout is related to the same physiological phenomenon that produces kidney stones.

NEAT PAIN-RELIEVING AND ANTI-INFLAMMATORY TREATMENT

1 or 2 drops lavender or geranium essential oil

1. If the inflamed area is painful to the touch, chill it with ice-cold water.
2. Using your fingertip, apply the undiluted lavender or geranium essential oil directly to the inflamed area.
3. Repeat this treatment once a day until the inflammation subsides.

WARM COMPRESS

2 drops basil essential oil
2 drops frankincense essential oil

1. Apply the undiluted basil and frankincense essential oils directly to the inflamed, painful area.
2. Follow the instructions in chapter 3 for making a warm compress (page 48).
3. Place the warm compress on the affected area.
4. Remove the compress when it cools to body temperature.
5. Repeat this treatment 2 or 3 times a day as necessary for relief from pain and inflammation.

Hair Loss

A certain amount of hair loss is normal—about 20 to 100 strands a day—but if you're losing more hair than that, natural remedies can play a role in slowing the process. As a bonus, these remedies help you improve the health of your scalp and eliminate the chemical buildup associated with commercial shampoos and other hair products.

1 ounce jojoba carrier oil
5 drops cedarwood essential oil
5 drops lavender essential oil
5 drops rosemary essential oil
5 drops thyme essential oil

1. Pour the jojoba carrier oil into a small glass or ceramic bowl.
2. Add the cedarwood, lavender, rosemary, and thyme essential oils to the carrier oil, and stir to combine.
3. Pour this blend into the palm of your hand, and massage your scalp for 2 minutes, then rinse.
4. Repeat this treatment 3 or 4 times a week to minimize hair loss.

Hangover

When you tie one on at night, sometimes you have to pay for it the next morning. If so, you'll need plenty of rest, and you'll have to replace the fluids lost to alcohol's dehydrating effects. In addition, three essential oils—lavender, lemon, and peppermint—can help you get through the worst of the symptoms.

NEAT MORNING-AFTER SHOWER TREATMENT

6 drops peppermint essential oil

1. Put 3 drops of the undiluted peppermint essential oil on a wet washcloth.
2. Put the washcloth on the floor of your shower.
3. Turn the water on, and let the shower fill up with steam.
4. Step into the shower, or sit nearby if you can't stay on your feet, and breathe in the scent of the peppermint oil for 10 minutes.
5. Turn the water off.

6. Using a cotton ball, apply 1 drop of undiluted peppermint oil to one temple, 1 drop to the other temple, and 1 drop to the back of your neck for relief from a headache and nausea.

MORNING-AFTER DIFFUSER BLEND

10 drops lavender essential oil
10 drops peppermint essential oil

1. Add the lavender and peppermint essential oils to the water in your diffuser.
2. Turn the diffuser on, and let it run while you rest or nap.
3. Repeat this treatment as often as necessary to relieve your symptoms.

MORNING-AFTER CALMING BLEND

1 tablespoon carrier oil
8 drops lemon essential oil

1. Pour the carrier oil into a small glass or ceramic bowl.
2. Add the lemon essential oil to the carrier oil, and stir to combine.
3. Smooth this blend all over your body to relieve tension.

Hay Fever

See **Allergies (Seasonal)**, page 64.

Headache

Essential oils are some of the best and most effective remedies for headaches, as physicians already knew for hundreds of years before pharmaceuticals became the well-advertised remedies of choice. More recently, in a small-scale study with a double-blind, placebo-controlled, randomized cross-over design, researchers obtained significant reduction in headache pain from topical use of peppermint essential oil combined with ethanol (alcohol).[23]

1 ounce vodka
5 drops peppermint essential oil

1. Pour the vodka into a small glass or ceramic bowl.
2. Add the peppermint essential oil to the vodka, and stir to combine.
3. Using a cotton ball, apply this blend with broad strokes all over your forehead, your temples, and the back of your neck.
4. With your eyes closed, do your best to relax until the pain subsides.

COLD PACK

1 cup refrigerated water
5 drops peppermint essential oil

1. Pour the refrigerated water into a glass or ceramic bowl or low basin.
2. Add the peppermint essential oil to the water.
3. Follow the instructions in chapter 3 for making a cold pack (page 46).
4. Place the cold pack on your forehead.
5. Keep the cold pack in place until it warms to body temperature.
6. Repeat this treatment as often as needed to reduce headache pain.

EMERGENCY NEAT TREATMENT

3 drops peppermint essential oil

Using a cotton ball, apply 1 drop of undiluted peppermint essential oil to one temple, 1 drop to the other temple, and 1 drop to the back of your neck until you're able to use a more complete treatment.

Hemorrhoids

Hemorrhoids, a fairly common ailment, feel much worse than they actually are—an important thing to remember when they're inflamed. Several essential oils can offer pain relief.

3 drops helichrysum essential oil
3 drops lavender essential oil

1. Run a warm bath.
2. Add the helichrysum and lavender essential oils to the bathwater.
3. Soak until the water cools to body temperature.

2 drops frankincense essential oil

Using a cotton ball, apply the undiluted frankincense essential oil directly to the inflamed hemorrhoid for pain relief, or as a follow-up to cleansing with a flushable premoistened wipe.

Hiccups

Hiccups rarely last longer than a few minutes, but if they become uncomfortable, the trick to stopping them is to break their spasmodic cycle.

1 bottle peppermint essential oil

1. Open the bottle of peppermint essential oil.
2. Hold the bottle up to your nose, and inhale continuously for 10 seconds.
3. Repeat this treatment until the hiccups stop.

1 drop cypress essential oil
1 drop tarragon essential oil

1. Put the undiluted tarragon essential oil on one index finger.
2. Put the undiluted cypress essential oil on your other index finger.
3. Place both fingers against your esophagus (in the notch at the center of your throat).
4. Curl your fingers downward to apply the oils, and then quickly release them.

Hives

These itchy pink bumps and welts will usually go away on their own within 24 hours, but they're very uncomfortable while they're around. Here are some natural approaches to relieving the misery.

ANTI-ITCH BODY WASH

2 cups water
3 tablespoons baking soda
5 drops chamomile essential oil
2 drops peppermint essential oil

1. Pour the water into a glass or ceramic bowl.
2. Add the baking soda to the water along with the chamomile and peppermint essential oils, and stir to combine.
3. Pour ¼ cup of the solution into a second glass or ceramic bowl, and set it aside for use in the Anti-Itch Paste described next in this section.
4. Using a clean, soft washcloth, gently apply this body wash to skin affected by hives.
5. Repeat this treatment as necessary to relieve itching.

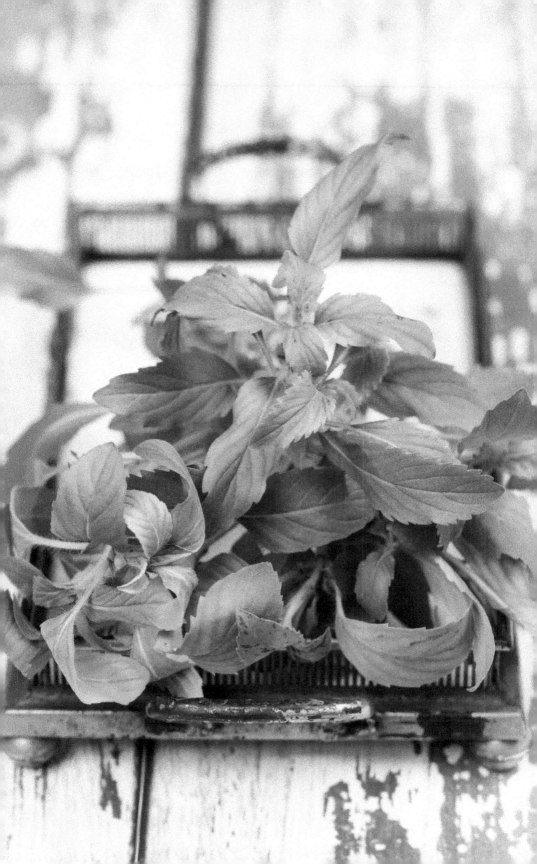

¼ cup Anti-Itch Body Wash (described earlier in this section)
3 tablespoons bentonite clay

1. Pour the Anti-Itch Body Wash into a small glass or ceramic bowl.
2. Add the clay, and stir to combine and form a paste.
3. Using your fingertips, apply this paste directly to skin affected by hives.
4. Leave the paste on for 45 minutes, and then gently wash it off.
5. Repeat this treatment as necessary to relieve itching.[24]

Hot Flashes

See **Menopause Symptoms**, page 140.

Hypertension

Essential oils are not a substitute for medication that your doctor may have prescribed for hypertension (better known as high blood pressure), but they can have a positive effect on your blood pressure by helping you manage stress.

DOCTOR'S ORDERS Always talk with your doctor before using any essential oil to make sure it won't interfere with medications you're taking for high blood pressure or other conditions.

DIFFUSER BLEND

1 drop bergamot essential oil
1 drop lavender essential oil
1 drop ylang-ylang essential oil

1. Add the bergamot, lavender, and ylang-ylang essential oils to the water in your diffuser.

2. Turn the diffuser on, and let it run for 15 minutes out of every hour in the evening.
3. For continuous treatment, place the diffuser next to your bed, and let it run it all night.

MASSAGE BLEND
....

½ ounce apricot kernel carrier oil
2 drops bergamot essential oil
2 drops frankincense essential oil
1 drop ylang-ylang essential oil

1. Pour the apricot kernel carrier oil into a small glass or ceramic bowl.
2. Add the bergamot, frankincense, and ylang-ylang essential oils to the carrier oil, and stir to combine.
3. Using your fingertips, apply this blend to your torso and back, and massage it into the skin to improve circulation and promote relaxation.
4. Repeat this treatment once a day, especially in the evening.

Indigestion
....

Indigestion can be caused by a number of things, including an unusually large meal, certain foods, medical conditions, a course of antibiotics, or use of other prescription medications. Whatever its causes, indigestion can keep you from getting a good night's sleep. Here's a bedtime remedy.

NEAT TREATMENT
....

3 or 4 drops peppermint essential oil

1. At bedtime, apply the undiluted peppermint essential oil to your pillow.
2. Breathe in the aroma overnight as you sleep to calm your stomach and promote general relaxation.

Ingrown Toenail

An ingrown toenail isn't just painful. It can also become an abscess and lead to even more serious complications. If you've had an ingrown toenail before and are familiar enough with the condition to be sure your nail is not infected, try relieving the pain with essential oils that have soothing and disinfectant properties.

WHEN TO SEE A DOCTOR If your toe is red, swollen, and painful to the touch, your ingrown toenail is probably infected. You need to see a doctor, who may prescribe an antibiotic and refer you to a podiatrist for further treatment. *See a doctor right away if you have diabetes and/or poor circulation or nerve damage in the affected foot or leg.*

NEAT BLEND

1 drop lavender essential oil
1 drop tea tree essential oil

1. Using a cotton ball, apply the undiluted essential oils directly to the ingrown toenail, being careful to swab the area where the toenail has grown into the skin.
2. Repeat this treatment 2 times a day until the nail grows out and the pain subsides.

ANTISEPTIC BLEND

1 ounce olive carrier oil
3 drops oregano essential oil

To make the blend

1. Pour the olive carrier oil into a small glass or ceramic bowl.
2. Add the oregano essential oil to the carrier oil, and stir to combine.
3. Pour the blend into a dark-colored glass bottle that closes tightly, and store the bottle in the refrigerator between uses.

To use the blend

1. Using a cotton swab, apply the blend to the affected toenail.
2. Repeat this treatment 3 times a day until the nail grows out.

Insect Bites

Mosquitoes, gnats, chiggers, and other biting insects can inflict a misery of itching, and few over-the-counter remedies are particularly effective against it. But essential oils with anti-itching properties can deliver relief in minutes and even leach out the toxins that a bite leaves behind.

NEAT ANTI-ITCHING TREATMENT

1 drop lavender or tea tree essential oil

1. Using a cotton ball, apply the undiluted lavender essential oil directly to the bite.
2. Repeat this treatment as necessary to relieve itching.

HEALING PASTE

1 tablespoon bentonite clay
2 teaspoons distilled water
1 teaspoon calendula carrier oil
12 drops lavender oil
5 drops chamomile oil

To make the paste

1. Put the clay in a dark-colored glass jar that closes tightly.
2. Gradually add the distilled water and calendula carrier oil to the clay, and stir to combine.
3. Add the lavender and chamomile essential oils to the mixture, and stir to create a thick paste. (If it's too thick, thin it with a little more distilled water.)
4. Close the jar tightly, and store it in the refrigerator between uses. (If the paste dries out in the jar, add a little distilled water.)

To use the paste

1. Using your fingertips, apply the paste directly to the insect bite, and allow it to dry.
2. When the paste dries, brush it off.
3. Repeat this treatment as often as necessary for relief from painful bites.[25]

BLOCK THAT BITE When it comes to mosquitoes, citronella essential oil has been known for centuries to be an effective repellent.[26] But lately catnip has been getting into the act, too—catnip essential oil contains nepetalactone, a natural chemical discovered to be so effective against biting insects that it vastly outperforms DEET, the notorious toxin found in many commercial insect repellents.[27]

Insomnia

Getting enough sleep is an important priority for everyone. Essential oils can do a lot to break down the barriers to restful sleep.

BEDTIME BATH BLEND

½ cup milk
3 drops lavender essential oil
2 drops Roman chamomile essential oil
1 drop clary sage essential oil
1 drop marjoram essential oil
1 drop ylang-ylang essential oil

1. Pour the milk into a small glass or ceramic bowl.
2. Add the lavender, Roman chamomile, clary sage, marjoram, and ylang-ylang essential oils to the milk, and stir to combine.
3. Run a warm bath.
4. Add this blend to the bathwater.
5. Soak until the water cools to body temperature, and then dry off and slip into bed.[28]

Irritable Bowel Syndrome

Like people who have colitis and Crohn's disease, people with irritable bowel syndrome (IBS) suffer from cramping, diarrhea, vomiting, and the nutritional deficiencies that can result. But IBS is not an autoimmune disease, so it's possible to find remedies that can help keep the digestive system in a state of relative calm.

ANTI-CRAMPING BATH BLEND

¼ cup of milk
3 drops basil essential oil
3 drops marjoram essential oil
3 drops peppermint essential oil

1. Pour the milk into a small glass or ceramic bowl.
2. Add the basil, marjoram, and peppermint essential oils to the milk, and stir to combine.
3. Run a warm bath.
4. Add the milk mixture to the bathwater.
5. Soak until the water cools to body temperature.
6. Repeat this treatment as often as necessary to relieve cramping.

MASSAGE BLEND

5 milliliters jojoba carrier oil
3 drops basil essential oil
3 drops marjoram essential oil
3 drops rosemary essential oil

1. Pour the jojoba carrier oil into a small glass or ceramic bowl.
2. Add the basil, marjoram, and rosemary essential oils to the carrier oil, and stir to combine.
3. Using your fingertips, apply this blend to your abdomen, and massage it into the skin.
4. Repeat this treatment as often as necessary to aid elimination and relieve cramping.

3 drops eucalyptus essential oil

2 drops Roman chamomile essential oil

2 drops neroli essential oil

2 drops peppermint essential oil

1. Add the eucalyptus, chamomile, neroli, and peppermint essential oils to the water in your diffuser.
2. Turn the diffuser on, and let it run for 15 minutes of every hour, until your system returns to normal.

Jock Itch

Jock itch results from a fungal infection. Over-the-counter preparations designed to control the infection will work, but it can take weeks for the rash and itching to disappear completely. Essential oils can help you manage the symptoms of jock itch and feel more comfortable while you wait for the infection to clear up.

ANTIFUNGAL WASH

1 cup water

2 drops cypress essential oil

1. Pour the water into a glass or ceramic bowl.
2. Add the cypress essential oil, and stir to combine.
3. Using a clean, soft washcloth, apply this blend to the area affected by jock itch.
4. Dry the area completely with a blow-dryer turned to the lowest setting.
5. Repeat this treatment as often as necessary to let the antifungal properties of the cypress oil work on the infection.

1 teaspoon olive carrier oil
2 drops lavender essential oil
2 drops tea tree oil

1. Pour the olive carrier oil into a small glass or ceramic bowl.
2. Add the lavender and tea tree essential oils to the carrier oil, and stir to combine.
3. Using your fingertips, apply this blend to the area affected by jock itch 2 times a day, in the morning and at bedtime.
4. Wear clean cotton underwear during the day, and repeat this treatment until the infection begins to heal.

Joint Inflammation (Injury-Related)

An injury—from playing a sport, taking a fall, or being involved in an automobile accident—can leave one or more of your joints swollen and painful. The first order of business after an injury is to immobilize the affected joint and treat the inflammation so healing can begin as soon as possible.

COLD PACK

1 pint refrigerated water
2 drops German chamomile essential oil (other choices: basil, eucalyptus, frankincense, ginger, lavender, myrrh, peppermint, or wintergreen)

1. Pour the refrigerated water into a glass or ceramic bowl or low basin.
2. Add the German chamomile essential oil to the water.
3. Follow the instructions in chapter 3 for making a cold pack (page 46).

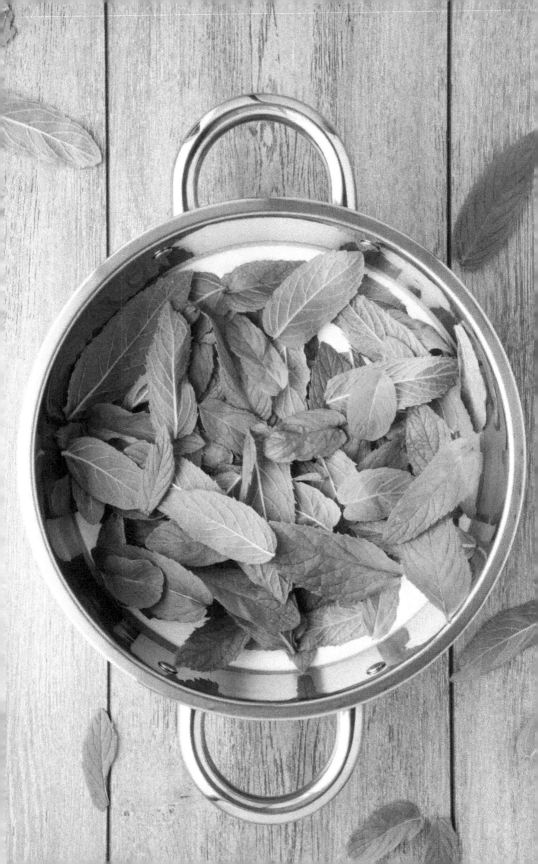

4. Keep the cold pack in place over the inflamed joint, replacing the water with freshly refrigerated water as necessary.
5. Repeat this treatment as necessary to reduce inflammation and pain.

Leg Cramps

A leg cramp that wakes you up in the middle of the night may be caused by an overused muscle, a mineral deficiency, or the effects of dehydration. However a leg cramp starts, you can have this massage blend at your fingertips to make it stop and let you to go back to sleep.

MASSAGE BLEND

1 tablespoon carrier oil
1 tablespoon basil essential oil
1 tablespoon juniper berry essential oil
1 tablespoon marjoram essential oil

To make the blend

1. Pour the carrier oil into a small glass or ceramic bowl.
2. Add the basil, juniper berry, and marjoram essential oils to the carrier oil, and stir to combine.
3. Pour this blend into a dark-colored glass bottle that closes tightly, and keep it at your bedside.

To use the blend

1. For a sudden leg cramp, pour a few drops of the blend into the palm of your hand, and massage it into the skin over the cramped muscle.
2. For chronic leg cramps, pour a few drops of the blend into the palm of your hand, and massage it into the skin over the cramped muscles 3 times a day to relieve pain and restore flexibility.
3. After each rub, follow the instructions in chapter 3 for making a warm compress (page 48), and apply the compress to help the oils be absorbed into your skin and loosen tight muscles.

Lice

Head lice are common among children from every background, at every school, and in every part of the country. With lice comes the need to alter a child's daily routine to include processes for removing lice and preventing their return.

PRELIMINARY OIL TREATMENT

Olive or sweet almond carrier oil

1. Before using any essential oils, coat the child's hair with olive carrier oil.
2. Using an ordinary comb, separate the hair into sections. While you're working on one section, hold other sections out of the way with hair clips.
3. Using a lice comb (available at a pharmacy), go through the child's hair to find the lice. Remove the lice with the comb, and discard them.
4. Wash the hair with the child's regular shampoo. Rinse, and then wash and rinse the hair again.
5. Dry the hair with a towel, which should immediately be washed.
6. Wash the ordinary comb, lice comb, hair clips, and any other tools you've used by soaking them in vinegar for 30 minutes.
7. Repeat this routine once a day for 1 week.
8. Continue to comb out the child's hair with the lice comb for another 2 weeks, taking care to wash the lice comb and other tools by soaking them in vinegar for 30 minutes after each use.

SAFETY REMINDER When blending essential oils for a child, use half the strength you would use for yourself: a 1 percent dilution instead of the usual 2 percent dilution for an adult.

OVERNIGHT DELOUSING BLEND

2 ounces olive carrier oil
15 to 20 drops lavender or tea tree essential oil

1. Pour the olive carrier oil into a small glass or ceramic bowl.
2. Add the lavender essential oil to the carrier oil, and stir to combine.
3. Using a cotton ball, apply this blend to the child's scalp at bedtime, and leave it on overnight (at least 12 hours).
4. In the morning, comb through the child's hair with the lice comb to find the lice. Remove the lice with the comb, and discard them.
5. Shampoo the child's hair as usual.
6. Dry the hair with a towel, which should immediately be washed.
7. Wash the lice comb and any other tools you've used by soaking them in vinegar for 30 minutes.

OVERNIGHT LICE-PREVENTION SPRAY

4 ounces rubbing alcohol
15 to 20 drops lavender or tea tree essential oil

1. Pour the rubbing alcohol into a small glass spray bottle.
2. Add the lavender essential oil to the rubbing alcohol, and shake well to blend.
3. Spray this blend on the child's hair once a day, at bedtime, for 2 weeks.
4. In the morning, comb through the child's hair with the lice comb to find and remove any remaining lice and to check for their reappearance.
5. Shampoo the child's hair as usual.
6. Dry the hair with a towel, which should immediately be washed.
7. Wash the lice comb and any other tools you've used by soaking them in vinegar for 30 minutes.

Menopause Symptoms

The hormonal changes that take place during menopause can throw a middle-aged woman's life into quiet chaos. Hot flashes are probably the best-known menopausal symptom, but they're only the tip of the melting iceberg. Some essential oils balance the hormones and moderate this troublesome symptom. Others offer cooling relief. Here are some remedies that can help with hot flashes and other physical and emotional challenges of the menopausal years.

COOLING SPRITZ

3 ounces spring water
1 ounce witch hazel extract
8 drops clary sage essential oil
8 drops peppermint essential oil
8 drops Roman chamomile essential oil

1. Pour the spring water into a 4-ounce glass spray bottle.
2. Add the witch hazel extract along with the clary sage, peppermint, and Roman chamomile essential oils to the water, and shake well to blend.
3. Use this blend to give yourself a spray when you feel a hot flash coming on.[29]

NEAT COOLING TREATMENT

1 drop clary sage essential oil
1 drop geranium essential oil
1 drop peppermint essential oil

1. Using your fingertip, apply the undiluted clary sage, geranium, and peppermint essential oils to the back of your neck while getting dressed in the morning.
2. Repeat this treatment as necessary during the day to relieve hot flashes.

ROLL-ON BLEND FOR NIGHT SWEATS

8 drops lavender essential oil
6 drops clary sage essential oil
4 drops bergamot essential oil
4 drops cedarwood essential oil
4 drops geranium essential oil
4 drops ylang-ylang essential oil
3 drops carrot seed essential oil

3 drops fennel essential oil

3 drops palma rosa essential oil

1. Transfer the lavender, clary sage, bergamot, cedarwood, geranium, ylang-ylang, carrot seed, fennel, and palma rosa essential oils to a dark-colored glass bottle with a roll-on applicator.
2. Roll this blend on the bottoms of your feet.
3. Repeat this treatment once a day, at bedtime.
4. Store the blend in the refrigerator between uses.

MOOD-STABILIZING BATH SALTS

3 cups sea salt

3 teaspoons coconut carrier oil

6 drops jasmine essential oil

6 drops neroli essential oil

6 drops Roman chamomile essential oil

To make the bath salts

1. Pour the sea salt into a ceramic or glass bowl.
2. Drizzle the coconut carrier oil over the salt 1 teaspoon at a time, mixing after each drizzle to prevent clumping.
3. Add the jasmine, neroli, and Roman chamomile essential oils to the salt mixture, and stir to combine.
4. Store the bath salts in a dark-colored glass jar that closes tightly.

To use the bath salts

1. Run a warm bath.
2. Add up to 1 cup of bath salts to the bathwater, swirling to make sure the salts are dissolved.
3. Soak for as long as you like.
4. Repeat this treatment as necessary to relieve moodiness.

HORMONE-BALANCING MASSAGE BLEND

1 teaspoon carrier oil

2 drops chamomile essential oil

2 drops jasmine essential oil

2 drops neroli essential oil

1. Pour the carrier oil into a small glass or ceramic bowl.
2. Add the chamomile, jasmine, and neroli essential oils to the carrier oil, and stir to combine.
3. Using your fingertips, apply this blend to your thighs, buttocks, back, and arms, massaging the oils into the deep tissues, which hold the highest concentrations of hormones.

Menstrual Cramps

In 2011, researchers in Korea found aromatherapy massage more effective than Tylenol in reducing the pain of menstrual cramps for adolescent girls.[30] Try this remedy for a natural alternative.

NEAT TREATMENT

5 to 10 drops clary sage essential oil

1. Using your fingertips, apply the undiluted clary sage essential oil to your lower abdomen and lower back.
2. Rub in a clockwise motion, and let the oil be absorbed through your skin.
3. Repeat this treatment no more than 2 times a day.

MASSAGE BLEND

1 teaspoon sweet almond carrier oil
2 drops clary sage essential oil
2 drops geranium essential oil
2 drops ginger essential oil
2 drops marjoram essential oil

1. Pour the sweet almond carrier oil into a small glass or ceramic bowl.
2. Add the clary sage, geranium, ginger, and marjoram essential oils to the carrier oil, and stir to combine.
3. Using your fingertips, apply this blend to your lower abdomen and lower back, rubbing in a clockwise motion.
4. Repeat no more than 2 times a day. If cramps are severe, follow up with a warm compress, described next in this section.

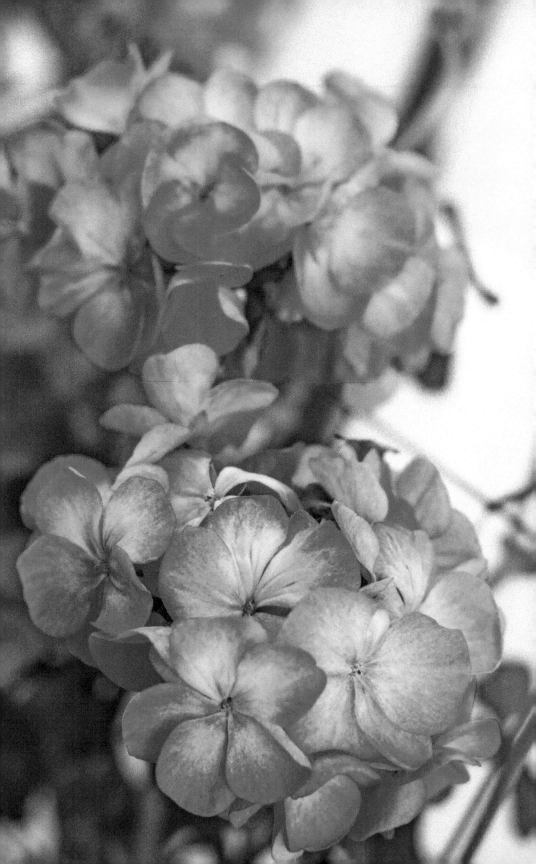

1 pint warm water
2 drops clary sage essential oil
2 drops geranium essential oil
2 drops ginger essential oil
2 drops marjoram essential oil

1. Follow the instructions in chapter 3 for making a warm compress (page 48).
2. Place the warm compress on the lower abdomen.
3. Remove the compress when it cools to body temperature.
4. Repeat this treatment as necessary to relieve pain.

Metabolism (Slow)

The right essential oils can be the key to raising your energy level or ramping up your metabolic rate so you can drop those extra pounds.

MASSAGE BLEND

1 tablespoon sweet almond carrier oil
3 drops grapefruit essential oil
3 drops lemon essential oil
2 drops cinnamon essential oil
2 drops ginger essential oil
2 drops peppermint essential oil

1. Pour the sweet almond carrier oil into a small glass or ceramic bowl.
2. Add the grapefruit, lemon, cinnamon, ginger, and peppermint essential oils to the carrier oil, and stir to combine.
3. Using your fingertips, apply this blend all over your body, and massage it into the skin.
4. Repeat this treatment 2 times a day, morning and night.

3 drops grapefruit essential oil
3 drops lemon essential oil
2 drops cinnamon essential oil
2 drops ginger essential oil
2 drops peppermint essential oil

1. Transfer the grapefruit, lemon, cinnamon, ginger, and peppermint essential oils into a glass or ceramic bowl, and stir to combine.
2. Pour this blend into a dark-colored glass bottle that closes tightly, and store the bottle in the refrigerator between uses.
3. Add 2 drops of this blend to the water in your diffuser.
4. Turn the diffuser on, place it next to your bed, and let it run overnight.

ENERGY SPRAY

12 ounces distilled water
1 tablespoon vodka
10 drops bergamot essential oil
10 drops grapefruit essential oil
10 drops sweet orange essential oil

1. Pour the distilled water into a 16-ounce glass spray bottle.
2. Add the vodka along with the bergamot, grapefruit, and sweet orange essential oils to the water, and shake well to blend.
3. Spray this blend around the room as often as you feel the need for an energy boost.

Migraine

A migraine is a particular kind of extremely painful headache that causes problems with vision and sensitivity to light, and is accompanied, in the worst cases, by nausea and vomiting. When the first symptoms appear, it can be helpful to regulate the body temperature so that blood vessels can achieve a dilated state in which the developing migraine can perhaps be arrested. For those who suffer from a specific, very severe type of migraine called a *cluster headache*, cayenne (capsaicin) can be used as a preventive treatment.

PREVENTIVE SOAK

1 quart warm water (110 degrees)
5 drops ginger essential oil
5 drops lavender essential oil

1. Pour the warm water into a glass or ceramic bowl or basin.
2. Add the ginger and lavender essential oils to the water.
3. At the first appearance of migraine symptoms, soak your hands and wrists in this solution for at least 3 minutes to rebalance your body's temperature, allow constricted blood vessels to relax, and possibly prevent a full-blown migraine from developing.

PREVENTIVE WARM COMPRESS

1 pint warm water
5 drops ginger essential oil
5 drops lavender essential oil

1. Follow the instructions in chapter 3 for making a warm compress (page 48).
2. Place the warm compress on your forehead.
3. Remove the compress when it cools to body temperature.
4. Repeat this treatment as necessary to arrest a developing migraine.

ANALGESIC/ANTI-INFLAMMATORY BLEND

1 tablespoon unscented hand lotion
5 drops cayenne essential oil

1. Pour the hand lotion into a small glass or ceramic bowl.
2. Add the cayenne essential oil to the lotion, and stir to combine.

3. Using your fingertips, smooth this blend onto your forehead and temples.
4. Repeat this treatment as necessary to dilate blood vessels and reduce pain.

TOO HOT TO HANDLE Do not use cayenne essential oil in undiluted form. It can be very irritating to the skin.

Moodiness

The whole point of aromatherapy is to bring calm, reason, and good health to your life. A number of mood-regulating essential oils—geranium, lavender, mandarin, neroli, and Roman chamomile, among others—can help you find your way back to your grounded center. Essential oils won't resolve a serious mood disorder or other psychological or psychiatric conditions, but they can boost your spirits and help you shake off a stressful day.

SPRITZ

2 ounces carrier oil
6 drops cinnamon essential oil
3 drops cedarwood essential oil
3 drops geranium essential oil

1. Pour the carrier oil into a small glass spray bottle.
2. Add the cinnamon, cedarwood, and geranium essential oils to the carrier oil, and shake well to blend.
3. Spray this blend around your room as an air freshener—and mood lightener.

MIST

4 ounces distilled water
4 drops jasmine essential oil
1 drop vanilla essential oil

1. Pour the distilled water into a small glass spray bottle.
2. Add the jasmine and vanilla essential oils to the water, and shake well to blend.
3. Use this blend as an after-shower spray for an uplifting scent all day long.

MOOD-BALANCING DIFFUSER BLEND

2 drops mandarin essential oil
2 drops neroli essential oil

1. Add the mandarin and neroli essential oils to the water in your diffuser.
2. Turn the diffuser on.
3. For continuous treatment, place the diffuser next to your bed, and let it run it all night.

MOOD-BALANCING MASSAGE BLEND

1 tablespoon evening primrose carrier oil
2 drops geranium essential oil
2 drops lavender essential oil
2 drops Roman chamomile essential oil

1. Pour the evening primrose carrier oil into a small glass or ceramic bowl.
2. Add the geranium, lavender, and Roman chamomile essential oils to the carrier oil, and stir to combine.
3. Using your fingertips, apply this blend into areas of your body with dense tissue (hips, thighs, buttocks, and upper arms), and massage it into the skin.
4. Repeat this treatment as necessary to feel a positive, calming effect.

Motion Sickness

Motion sickness has little or nothing to do with the digestive system (which is why over-the-counter antinausea remedies don't help). It has to do with the inner ear and the conflict between what a traveler sees (the static inside of an automobile or aircraft) and what the traveler feels (forward motion and sometimes turbulence). For prevention and treatment of motion sickness, over-the-counter pharmaceuticals that contain dimenhydrinate are very effective, and so are prescription patches that contain scopolamine, but they can cause dry mouth and drowsiness. Here are some alternative approaches that use essential oils. They can't eliminate motion sickness altogether, but they can help control nausea.

NEAT TREATMENT

2 drops peppermint essential oil

1. Apply the undiluted peppermint essential oil to a handkerchief.
2. When you start to feel queasy, hold the handkerchief up to your nose, and inhale continuously for 10 seconds.
3. Repeat this treatment as necessary to quell nausea.

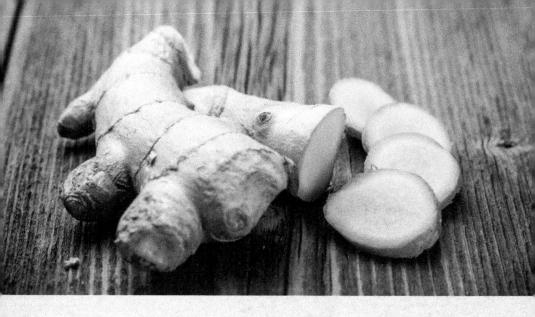

THE POWER OF GINGER
Alleviating Motion Sickness

Ginger has long been considered a remedy for motion sickness. In fact, ginger is the go-to choice among distributors of essential oils and practitioners of aromatherapy when it comes to recommending a remedy for motion sickness.

The scientific evidence for this choice is inconclusive, however: A study from 1988 found ginger to be an effective agent against motion sickness, but a study from 1991 found no such benefit from taking ginger.[31] But both studies used powdered ginger root, whose strength and effectiveness may not be directly comparable or relevant to the strength and effectiveness of highly concentrated ginger essential oil.

In any case, what aromatherapy practitioners suggest for motion sickness is to apply 2 or 3 drops of undiluted ginger essential oil to the back of the neck, the pulse points on the wrists, and the soles of the feet, or to put a drop of ginger in the palm of one hand, rub the hands together, cup them over the face, and inhale deeply.

Muscle Aches

When aches and pains threaten to put you out of action, try a cold pack or one of these blends.[32]

COLD PACK

1 pint refrigerated water
3 drops Roman chamomile essential oil
2 drops marjoram essential oil

1. Pour the refrigerated water into a glass or ceramic bowl or low basin.
2. Add the Roman chamomile and marjoram essential oils to the water.
3. Follow the instructions in chapter 3 for making a cold pack (page 46).
4. Place the cold pack on the affected area.
5. Keep the cold pack in place until it warms to body temperature.
6. Repeat this treatment as necessary to relieve pain.

MASSAGE BLEND

4 teaspoons carrier oil
4 drops lavender essential oil
4 drops rosemary essential oil
2 drops ginger essential oil

To make the blend

1. Pour the carrier oil into a small glass or ceramic bowl.
2. Add the lavender, rosemary, and ginger essential oils to the carrier oil, and stir to combine.
3. Pour the blend into a dark-colored glass bottle that closes tightly, and store the bottle in the refrigerator between uses.

To use the blend

1. Using your fingertips, apply a few drops of this blend to the affected muscle, and massage them into the skin.
2. Repeat this treatment as necessary to relieve pain.

4 teaspoons carrier oil
4 drops black pepper essential oil
4 drops cinnamon essential oil
2 drops ginger essential oil

To make the blend

1. Pour the carrier oil into a small glass or ceramic bowl.
2. Add the black pepper, cinnamon, and ginger essential oils to the carrier oil, and stir to combine.
3. Pour the blend into a dark-colored glass bottle that closes tightly, and store the bottle in the refrigerator between uses.

To use the blend

1. Using your fingertips, apply a few drops of this blend to the affected muscle, and massage them into the skin.
2. Repeat this treatment 2 times a day until symptoms improve.

Nausea

Whether you're suffering from a stomach virus, food poisoning, the symptoms of colitis, or the rigors of chemotherapy, nausea is inevitably disagreeable, but a number of essential oils can moderate nausea and have antiemetic (anti-vomiting) properties.

ANTINAUSEA DIFFUSER BLEND

2 drops basil essential oil
2 drops bergamot essential oil
2 drops chamomile essential oil

1. Add the basil, bergamot, and chamomile essential oils to the water in your diffuser.
2. Turn the diffuser on, and let it run for 15 minutes of every hour.
3. Repeat this treatment as necessary to relieve nausea.

3 drops bergamot essential oil
3 drops chamomile essential oil

1. Run a warm bath.
2. Add the bergamot and chamomile essential oils to the bathwater.
3. Inhale deeply, and soak until the water cools to body temperature.
4. Repeat this treatment as necessary to relieve nausea.

DAB-ON ANTINAUSEA BLEND

1 tablespoon jojoba carrier oil
2 drops ginger essential oil
2 drops nutmeg essential oil
2 drops wintergreen essential oil

1. Pour the jojoba carrier oil into a small glass or ceramic bowl.
2. Add the ginger, nutmeg, and wintergreen essential oils to the carrier oil, and stir to combine.
3. Using your fingertips, dab 1 to 3 drops of this blend behind your ears and on the skin around your navel.
4. Repeat this treatment once per hour until the nausea subsides.

NEAT INHALATION TREATMENT

1 bottle patchouli essential oil

1. Open the bottle of patchouli essential oil.
2. Hold the bottle up to your nose, and inhale continuously for 10 seconds.
3. Repeat this treatment every 10 minutes to relax the muscles and reduce the contractions that come with vomiting.

ANTIEMETIC BLEND

1 teaspoon jojoba carrier oil
4 drops patchouli essential oil

1. Pour the jojoba carrier oil into a small glass or ceramic bowl.

2. Add the patchouli essential oil to the carrier oil, and stir to combine.
3. Using your fingertips, dab 3 drops of this blend behind your ears and on the skin around your navel.
4. Follow the instructions in chapter 3 for making a warm compress (page 48).
5. Place the warm compress on your stomach.
6. Remove the compress when it cools to body temperature.
7. Repeat this treatment as necessary until the vomiting subsides.

Neck Stiffness

Maybe you slept in the wrong position, or maybe your neck is in knots because of stress at work or at home. The essential oils you use to relieve the stiffness will depend on what's causing it.

STRESS-FIGHTING BLEND

1 teaspoon carrier oil
2 drops lavender essential oil
2 drops peppermint essential oil

1. Pour the carrier oil into a small glass or ceramic bowl.
2. Add the lavender and peppermint essential oils to the carrier oil, and stir to combine.
3. Using your fingertips, apply this blend into the stiff muscles at the base of your neck and along your shoulders, and massage it into the skin.
4. Repeat this treatment as necessary to restore calm to your emotions and flexibility to the muscles of your neck.

ANTI-INFLAMMATORY BLEND

1 teaspoon carrier oil
2 drops basil essential oil

1. Pour the carrier oil into a small glass or ceramic bowl.
2. Add the basil essential oil to the carrier oil, and stir to combine.

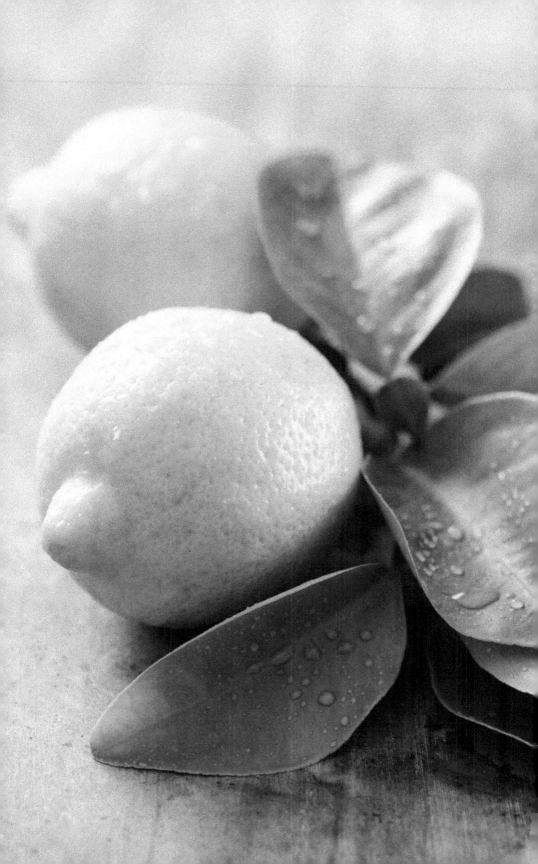

3. Using your fingertips, apply this blend into the inflamed areas of your neck and surrounding muscles, and massage it into the skin.
4. Repeat this treatment 2 or 3 times a day to relieve pain, spasms, and inflammation.

Nosebleed

Dry winter weather or the misery of a cold or flu can bring on a nosebleed, but the remedy couldn't be simpler.

NEAT BLEND

3 drops lemon essential oil
1 drop lavender essential oil

1. Pinch your nostrils together to stop the bleeding.
2. Apply the undiluted lemon and lavender essential oils to a tissue.
3. Hold the tissue up to your nose, and inhale.[33]

WHEN TO SEE A DOCTOR If you have suffered a blow to the nose, seek medical attention as soon as possible. Your nose may be broken and may need to be set and packed so it can heal properly.

COLD PACK

1 cup refrigerated water
3 drops lemon essential oil
1 drop lavender essential oil

1. Pour the refrigerated water into a glass or ceramic bowl or low basin.
2. Add the lemon and lavender essential oils to the water.
3. Follow the instructions in chapter 3 for making a cold pack (page 46).
4. Place the cold pack on your nose.

5. Keep the cold pack in place until it warms to body temperature or the nosebleed stops.
6. Repeat this treatment if the nosebleed has not stopped.

Oily Skin

If you're constantly fighting an oily sheen on your skin, you may be surprised to learn that essential oils that can help. Many have astringent properties and can remove excess oil during your daily cleansing while helping to balance out your skin's pH levels.

ASTRINGENT BLEND

1 teaspoon carrier oil

1 teaspoon frankincense essential oil (other choices: bergamot, clary sage, cypress, geranium, helichrysum, lavender, lemon, lemongrass, orange, patchouli, peppermint, Roman chamomile, rosemary, sandalwood, tea tree, or ylang-ylang)

1. Pour the carrier oil into a small glass or ceramic bowl.
2. Add the frankincense essential oil to the carrier oil, and stir to combine.
3. Using a cotton ball, apply the blend to your face after washing.
4. Repeat this treatment once a day.

NEAT BLEMISH-FIGHTING BLEND

2 drops tea tree essential oil
1 drop rosemary essential oil

1. Transfer the tea tree and rosemary essential oils to a small glass or ceramic bowl.
2. Using a cotton swab, apply the undiluted essential oils directly to blemishes.
3. Repeat this treatment 2 times a day until the blemishes disappear.

Osteoporosis

Osteoporosis (literally, porosity of the bones) is a progressive condition that often comes with advancing years and can lead to fractures of the wrist, hip, or vertebrae. Such an event can seriously compromise the ability to live independently. At this time, loss of bone density is not believed to be reversible, but certain essential oils may help slow the process.

MASSAGE BLEND

1 ounce evening primrose carrier oil
4 drops pine essential oil
3 drops eucalyptus essential oil
2 drops juniper berry essential oil
2 drops rosemary essential oil
2 drops sage essential oil

1. Pour the evening primrose carrier oil into a small glass or ceramic bowl.
2. Add the pine, eucalyptus, juniper berry, rosemary, and sage essential oils to the carrier oil, and stir to combine.
3. Using your fingertips, apply this blend to your spine, wrists, ankles, and all around your hips and pelvic region, and massage it into the skin.
4. Repeat this treatment once a day, in the morning or at bedtime.

BONING UP ON ESSENTIAL OILS A 2003 study found that essential oils containing thujone, camphor, and eucalyptol—pine oil in particular, but also eucalyptus, juniper berry, rosemary, and sage—inhibited loss of bone density in laboratory rats.[34] The results of the study are not conclusive for human beings, but that's no reason to keep from enjoying the benefits of these oils while research goes on. If you have osteoporosis, talk with your doctor about using essential oils, especially if you're taking prescription medication for this condition.

4 drops eucalyptus essential oil
4 drops pine essential oil

1. Add the eucalyptus and pine essential oils to the water in your diffuser.
2. Turn the diffuser on, and run it for 15 minutes of every hour.
3. For continuous treatment, place the diffuser next to your bed, and let it run all night.

Perspiration (Excess)

It's a natural fact that some of us just sweat more than others. Here are a couple of natural approaches to keeping profuse perspiration in check.

ROLL-ON BLEND FOR FEET

1 ounce carrier oil
48 drops lavender essential oil
36 drops clary sage essential oil
24 drops cypress essential oil

1. Pour the carrier oil into a small glass or ceramic bowl.
2. Add the lavender, clary sage, and cypress essential oils to the carrier oil, and stir to combine.
3. Transfer the blend to a dark-colored glass bottle with a roll-on applicator, and store it in the refrigerator between uses.
4. Roll the blend on the soles of your feet once a day, at bedtime.

DIFFUSER BLEND

4 drops clary sage essential oil
4 drops cypress essential oil

1. Add the clary sage and cypress essential oils to the water in your diffuser.

2. Turn the diffuser on.
3. For continuous treatment, place the diffuser next to your bed, and let it run overnight.

Poison Ivy

A walk in the woods can bring you into contact with poison ivy—and you may not even realize that you and this notorious plant have met until you break out in poison ivy's characteristic rash. Essential oils with antipruritic (anti-itch) properties can help you survive the worst of the misery.

URUSHIOL The rash associated with poison ivy comes from urushiol, an oil to which more than 90 percent of human beings are allergic. Urushiol can transfer from the poison ivy plant itself to shoes and clothing, a backpack, or an animal's fur and then onto your skin. Getting rid of urushiol takes multiple washings with a strong, oil-cutting soap. A good choice is Dawn, a liquid dishwashing detergent that is both strong and gentle enough to have been endorsed by the International Bird Rescue Research Center as the bird cleaner of choice after oil spills.[35]

ANTI-ITCH BLEND

1 teaspoon carrier oil

1 teaspoon lavender essential oil (other choices: peppermint, Roman chamomile, rose, or wintergreen)

1. Pour the carrier oil into a small glass or ceramic bowl.
2. Add the lavender essential oil to the carrier oil, and stir to combine.
3. Using a cotton ball, apply this blend to skin affected by poison ivy.
4. Repeat this treatment as necessary to relieve itching.

3 to 5 drops tea tree essential oil

1. Using a cotton ball, apply the undiluted tea tree oil to skin affected by poison ivy. If treating a large area, it might be necessary to use more essential oil.
2. Repeat this treatment as necessary to relieve itching.

See **Hives**, page 127

See **Hives**, page 127

Premenstrual Syndrome

Premenstrual syndrome (PMS) can include water retention, irritability, mood swings, breast tenderness, headaches, backache, and depression. All these symptoms can be relieved by essential oils used in a bath or for a massage.

3 cups sea salt
3 teaspoons jojoba carrier oil
6 drops clary sage essential oil
6 drops marjoram essential oil
3 drops angelica essential oil

To make the bath salts

1. Pour the sea salt into a ceramic or glass bowl.
2. Drizzle the jojoba carrier oil over the salt 1 teaspoon at a time, mixing after each drizzle to prevent clumping.
3. Add the clary sage, marjoram, and angelica essential oils to the salt, and stir to combine.
4. Store the bath salts in a dark-colored glass jar that closes tightly.

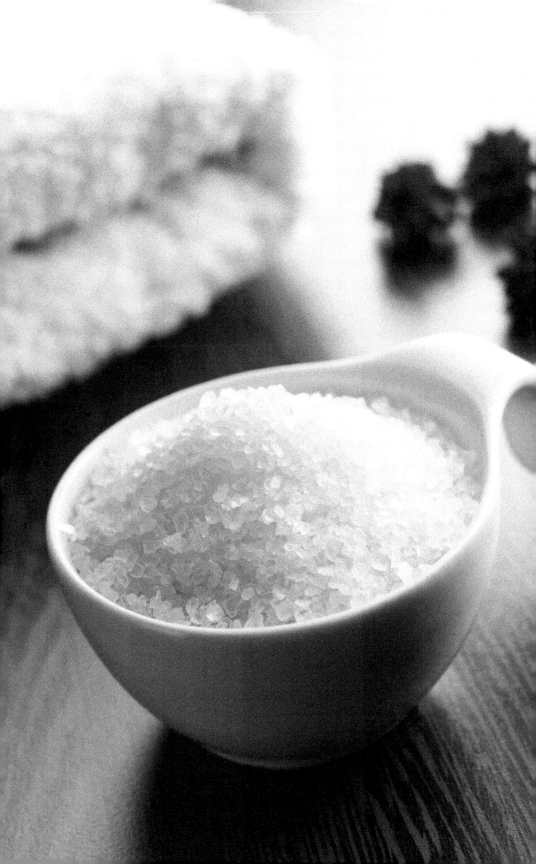

To use the bath salts

1. Run a warm bath.
2. Add ½ teaspoon of the bath salts to the running bathwater, swirling to make sure the salts are dissolved.
3. Soak for as long as you like.
4. Repeat this treatment as necessary to relieve PMS.

PMS MASSAGE BLEND
....

2 ounces carrier oil
4 drops angelica essential oil
4 drops chamomile essential oil
4 drops clary sage essential oil
4 drops geranium essential oil
4 drops marjoram essential oil

To make the blend

1. Pour the carrier oil into a small glass or ceramic bowl.
2. Add the angelica, chamomile, clary sage, geranium, and marjoram essential oils to the carrier oil, and stir to combine.
3. Pour the blend into a dark-colored glass bottle that closes tightly, and store the bottle in the refrigerator between uses.

To use the blend

1. Using your fingertips, apply this blend to your thighs, buttocks, back, and upper arms, massaging the oils into the deep tissues, which hold the highest concentrations of hormones.
2. Repeat this treatment once a day until symptoms are relieved.

Prostatitis

The symptoms of prostatitis include pain, inflammation, difficulty with urination, and lower back pain. Essential oils can't replace medical treatment when it's needed, but they can ease the symptoms.

1 ounce milk

3 drops sandalwood essential oil

1. Pour the milk into a small glass or ceramic bowl.
2. Add the sandalwood essential oil to the milk, and stir to combine.
3. Run a warm bath.
4. Add the blend to the bathwater.
5. Soak until the water cools to body temperature.
6. Repeat this treatment once a day until symptoms improve.

MASSAGE BLEND
....

1 teaspoon carrier oil

½ teaspoon German chamomile essential oil

½ teaspoon eucalyptus essential oil

1. Pour the carrier oil into a small glass or ceramic bowl.
2. Add the chamomile and eucalyptus essential oils to the carrier oil, and stir to combine.
3. Using your fingertips, apply this blend to the lower back and abdomen, and massage it into the skin.
4. Repeat this treatment 2 times a day until symptoms improve.

Psoriasis

In psoriasis, new skin cells are produced faster than usual, so the skin develops patches of new skin that are covered with old, dead skin flakes. Essential oils can help with the symptoms, but it may take some time.

SOOTHING BLEND
....

1 teaspoon carrier oil

3 drops patchouli essential oil

3 drops Roman chamomile essential oil

2 drops lavender essential oil

2 drops tea tree essential oil

1. Pour the carrier oil into a small glass or ceramic bowl.
2. Add the patchouli, Roman chamomile, lavender, and tea tree essential oils to the carrier oil, and stir to combine.
3. Using your fingertips, apply this blend to skin affected by psoriasis.
4. Repeat this treatment 2 times a day until symptoms improve.

1 teaspoon jojoba carrier oil
3 drops helichrysum essential oil
3 drops rose essential oil

1. Pour the jojoba carrier oil into a small glass or ceramic bowl.
2. Add the helichrysum and rose essential oils to the carrier oil, and stir to combine.
3. Using your fingertips, apply this blend to skin affected by psoriasis.
4. Repeat this treatment 2 times a day until symptoms improve.

Restless Leg Syndrome

Restless leg syndrome, considered a sleep disorder because it can wake a person up in the middle of the night, is the sensation that the skin is crawling as nerves misfire and the leg kicks involuntarily. Here are some remedies that can help with this condition.

MASSAGE BLEND

1 teaspoon grape seed, olive, or sweet almond carrier oil
4 drops Roman chamomile essential oil
4 drops lavender essential oil

1. Pour the grape seed carrier oil into a small glass or ceramic bowl.
2. Add the chamomile and lavender essential oils to the carrier oil, and stir to combine.

3. Using your fingertips, rub this blend into the skin of the legs at bedtime.
4. Repeat this treatment once a day until symptoms improve.

1 ounce milk
3 drops neroli or ylang-ylang essential oil

1. Run a warm bath.
2. Pour the milk into a small cup with a spout (like a measuring cup).
3. Add the neroli essential oil to the milk, and stir to combine.
4. Pour the blend into a warm bath.
5. Soak in the tub for 15 to 20 minutes before bed.
6. Repeat this treatment once a day.

Ringworm

A ring-shaped skin rash gives this fungal infection its name, though worms are not involved in any way. It appears as a dry, scaly inner ring with a red outer ring, which is the part that may be growing and spreading. This highly contagious infection easily passes to humans from pets.

ANTIFUNGAL BLEND

1 teaspoon jojoba or olive carrier oil
1 teaspoon lemongrass essential oil
1 teaspoon tea tree essential oil

1. Pour the jojoba carrier oil into a small glass or ceramic bowl.
2. Add the lemongrass and tea tree essential oils to the carrier oil, and stir to combine.
3. Using your fingertips, apply the blend directly to the infected area.
4. Repeat this treatment 2 times a day until the rash is no longer present. This may take several weeks.

ESSENTIAL OILS FOR APHRODISIAC BLENDS

Arousing Aromas

....

Blend three or four of these scents, at the very most. If you mix more, you'll get a heady blend that could prove overpowering—and not in a good way.

Citrus   Grapefruit, lemon, lime, mandarin, neroli, petitgrain, sweet orange, and tangerine add sweetness to a blend and make spicier oils a little less pungent.

Conifers   Balsam fir, cedarwood, cypress, fir needle, pine, scotch pine, and spruce add a fresh, tangy, natural scent that may be a turn-on for the rugged outdoorsman or outdoorswoman in your life.

Exotics   Ambrette seed, amyris, fennel, patchouli, sandalwood, star anise, vanilla, and vetiver contribute earthiness, richness, and the sense of another time and place.

Florals   Bergamot, geranium, jasmine, lavender, palma rosa, Roman chamomile, rose, rosewood, and ylang-ylang add sweetness and transporting light notes.

Mints   Chocolate peppermint, spearmint, and peppermint brighten the scent and add crispness.

Spices   Allspice, black pepper, cardamom, cinnamon, clove, coriander, frankincense, ginger, myrrh, and nutmeg are sensitizing and may need some tempering from citrus.

Sexual Dysfunction (Low Sex Drive)

No substance on earth will magically arouse someone who does not want to be aroused, but some essential oils can help create and build the mood in you or a willing partner.

EROTIC DIFFUSION

3 drops clove essential oil
3 drops sweet orange essential oil
3 drops vetiver essential oil

1. Add the clove, sweet orange, and vetiver essential oils to the water in your diffuser.
2. Turn the diffuser on, and allow it to run until the scent is noticeable (about 15 minutes).
3. Repeat this treatment in an hour, if you wish.

EROTIC MASSAGE BLEND

1 ounce jojoba or sweet almond carrier oil
2 drops essential oil from the conifers list
2 drops essential oil from the mint list
2 drops essential oil from the spice list

1. Pour the jojoba carrier oil into a small glass or ceramic bowl.
2. Add the conifer, mint, and spice essential oils to the carrier oil, and stir to combine.
3. Pour the combined oils into a small, dark-colored glass bottle.
4. Pour a few drops into your palm, and massage it into your partner's skin.

Sinus Pressure

The pressure that builds up in your sinuses when you have a cold can turn into a sinus infection, which can lead to an ear infection and other issues fairly quickly. Fight the congestion to avoid infection.

1 pint hot water
3 drops tea tree essential oil
1 drop eucalyptus essential oil

1. Pour the hot water into a glass or ceramic bowl.
2. Add the tea tree and eucalyptus essential oils to the water (they will remain on the water's surface).
3. Drape a towel over your head in such a way that it is also draped closely over the bowl.
4. Bend to hold your face over the bowl, and breathe deeply. *Keep your eyes closed.*
5. Remain in this position until the water cools, periodically lifting one side of the towel to take a breath of fresh air.
6. Repeat this treatment 3 times a day until the sinus pressure clears.

Skin Tags

Doctors really have no idea why people develop skin tags. The tags are harmless and will not become cancerous, but they can be annoying.

DAB-ON TREATMENT

1 teaspoon coconut carrier oil
5 drops oregano essential oil
1 drop peppermint essential oil

1. Pour the coconut carrier oil into a small glass or ceramic bowl.
2. Add the oregano and peppermint essential oils to the carrier oil, and stir to combine.
3. Using a cotton swab, dab the blend on your skin tags.
4. Repeat this treatment every night until the skin tags turn black and fall off (2 to 3 weeks).

1 teaspoon coconut carrier oil
3 drops frankincense essential oil
1 drop peppermint essential oil

1. Pour the coconut carrier oil into a small glass or ceramic bowl.
2. Add the frankincense and peppermint essential oils to the carrier oil, and stir to combine.
3. Using a cotton swab, dab the blend on your skin tags in the morning.
4. Repeat this treatment every morning until the skin tags turn black and fall off (2 to 3 weeks).

NEAT TREATMENT

2 drops jojoba or sweet almond carrier oil
1 drop clove, lemon, or oregano essential oil

1. With your fingertip or a cotton swab, rub the jojoba carrier oil on the skin around the skin tags (to protect the surrounding skin).
2. Place 1 drop of clove essential oil on a cotton swab, and brush the essential oil directly onto the skin tags.
3. Repeat this treatment once a day until the skin tags turn black and fall off (2 to 3 weeks).

Sore Throat

A seasonal cold, a strep infection, or an afternoon spent cheering for your favorite team can cause a sore throat. Calming the pain is the top priority.

WRAP

2 cups hot water
2 drops bergamot essential oil
2 drops lavender essential oil
1 drop tea tree essential oil

1. Pour the hot water into a medium glass or ceramic bowl.
2. Add the bergamot, lavender, and tea tree essential oils to the water.
3. Soak a soft towel or flannel cloth in the water.
4. Wring out the towel and wrap it around your neck
5. Cover it with a dry towel to hold in the heat, but make sure it's not so hot that it becomes uncomfortable.
6. Remove the wrap when it cools to body temperature.
7. Repeat this treatment as needed throughout the day until your throat is no longer sore.[36]

Spider Bite

If you know that the spider that bit you is not poisonous, you can treat the bite to reduce swelling and itching. If you are in an area in which the bite could be from a black widow or a brown recluse spider, seek emergency medical treatment.

ITCH-RELIEVING BLEND

1 teaspoon rubbing alcohol
3 drops lavender essential oil
2 drops Roman chamomile essential oil

1. Pour the alcohol into a small glass or ceramic bowl.
2. Add the lavender and Roman chamomile essential oils to the alcohol, and stir to combine.
3. Using a cotton ball, apply the blend to the spider bite.
4. Repeat this treatment up to 5 times a day until the swelling and itching are reduced.

Spider Veins

See **Blood Vessels (Broken)**, page 76

Splinter

Many splinters can be extracted with tweezers, but some penetrate deeply into the skin and need a little extra help to come to the surface. Essential oil can do the work for you without the pain of a needle.

NEAT TREATMENT

1 or 2 drops clove or lavender essential oil

1. Using your fingertip, apply the undiluted clove essential oil directly to the site of the splinter.
2. Wait 10 minutes, and then apply another drop if the splinter has not emerged.
3. When the splinter rises, use tweezers to remove it—or just let it slip out and brush it away.

Sprain

When a sudden twist of your knee, wrist, or ankle sends a painful shock through your limb and the area begins to swell, there's a good chance that you have a sprain. Start by elevating the injured area above your heart, applying ice or a cold pack for 20 minutes every three to four hours, and compressing the area with an elastic bandage.

HEALING BLEND FOR A SPRAIN WITH A BRUISE

1 teaspoon olive or sweet almond carrier oil
4 drops helichrysum essential oil

1. Pour the olive carrier oil into a small glass or ceramic bowl.
2. Add the helichrysum essential oil to the carrier oil, and stir to combine.
3. Using your fingertips, apply the blend to the area around the sprain, and massage it into the skin, especially wherever you see discoloration.
4. Repeat this treatment 2 times a day until the bruise fades.

1 teaspoon carrier oil
2 drops cypress essential oil
2 drops pine essential oil
2 drops spruce essential oil

1. Pour the carrier oil into a small glass or ceramic bowl.
2. Add the cypress, pine, and spruce essential oils to the carrier oil, and stir to combine.
3. Using your fingertips, apply the blend to the affected area, and massage it into the skin.
4. Wrap the area with an elastic bandage (firmly, but not tightly enough to cut off circulation).
5. Apply an ice or a cold pack.
6. Repeat this treatment every 3 to 4 hours until the swelling subsides.

NEAT MINT TREATMENT

2 drops peppermint or wintergreen essential oil

1. Using your fingertips, apply the undiluted peppermint essential oil to the affected area.
2. Alternately, add the peppermint essential oil to the healing blend described earlier in this section before massaging the blend into the injury.
3. Repeat this treatment 2 or 3 times a day until the pain subsides.

Stress and Tension

You may already be using your essential oils to treat symptoms of stress and tension, such as headaches, muscle aches, indigestion, and insomnia. Essential oils give you the opportunity to treat the feelings of stress that may be causing them.

2 ounces sweet almond carrier oil
10 drops lavender essential oil
6 drops Roman chamomile essential oil
4 drops sandalwood essential oil
4 drops ylang-ylang essential oil
1 drop neroli essential oil

1. Pour the sweet almond carrier oil into a small glass or ceramic bowl.
2. Add the lavender, Roman chamomile, sandalwood, ylang-ylang, and neroli essential oils to the carrier oil, and stir to combine.
3. Pour the blend into a dark-colored glass bottle that closes tightly, and store the bottle in the refrigerator between uses.
4. Using your fingertips, apply this blend to the affected area, and massage it into the skin.
5. Repeat this treatment once a day as needed.

BATH BLEND

4 ounces sweet almond carrier oil
20 drops lavender essential oil
12 drops Roman chamomile essential oil
8 drops sandalwood essential oil
8 drops ylang-ylang essential oil
2 drops neroli essential oil

1. Pour the sweet almond carrier oil into a small glass or ceramic bowl.
2. Add the lavender, Roman chamomile, sandalwood, ylang-ylang, and neroli essential oils to the carrier oil, and stir to combine.
3. Pour the blend into a dark-colored glass bottle that closes tightly, and store the bottle in the refrigerator between uses.
4. Run a warm bath. While the water is running, add 1 to 2 teaspoons of the blend to the tub.
5. Soak for at least 15 minutes, or until you feel less tense.

....

10 drops lavender essential oil

6 drops chamomile essential oil

4 drops sandalwood essential oil

4 drops ylang-ylang essential oil

1 drop neroli essential oil

1. Add the lavender, chamomile, sandalwood, ylang-ylang, and neroli essential oils to the water in your diffuser.
2. Turn the diffuser on, and allow it to run for at least 15 minutes.
3. Repeat this treatment 2 times a day until you feel more relaxed.

SPRAY
....

2 ounces distilled or filtered water

10 drops lavender essential oil

6 drops chamomile essential oil

4 drops sandalwood essential oil

4 drops ylang-ylang essential oil

1 drop neroli essential oil

1. Pour the water into a glass spray bottle.
2. Add the lavender, chamomile, sandalwood, ylang-ylang, and neroli essential oils to the water, and shake well to blend.
3. Spritz the blend in any room in your home, as often as you like, until you feel more relaxed.[37]

Stretch Marks

To help restore elasticity, heal damaged skin cells, and accelerate the growth of new cells, essential oils can be used on the pink or brown lines that appear on the abdomen, buttocks, hips, or breasts.

RUB
......

2 tablespoons sweet almond carrier oil

1 tablespoon wheat germ carrier oil

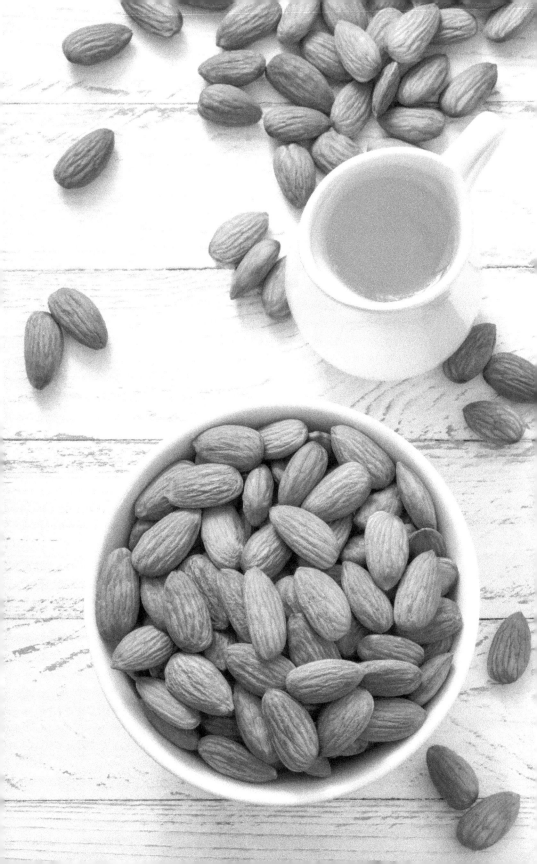

5 drops carrot carrier oil

10 drops borage seed essential oil

7 drops rose essential oil

6 drops lavender essential oil

5 drops tangerine essential oil

1. Pour the sweet almond, wheat germ, and carrot carrier oils into a small glass or ceramic bowl.
2. Add the borage seed, rose, lavender, and tangerine essential oils to the carrier oils, and stir to combine.
3. Pour the blend into a dark-colored glass bottle that closes tightly, and store the bottle in the refrigerator between uses.
4. Using your fingertips, apply a small amount to the stretch marks, and massage it into the skin.
5. Repeat this treatment once a day until the marks fade.[38]

1 ounce cocoa butter

12 drops tangerine essential oil

4 drops jasmine essential oil

1. Place the cocoa butter in a small glass or ceramic bowl.
2. Add the tangerine and jasmine essential oils to the cocoa butter, and stir to combine.
3. Pour the blend into a dark-colored glass bottle that closes tightly, and store the bottle in the refrigerator between uses.
4. Using your fingertips, apply a small amount to your stretch marks, and massage it into the skin.
5. Repeat this treatment 2 times a day until the marks fade.[39]

Sunburn

Even if you're scrupulous about wearing sunscreen whenever you go outside, once in a while you may find yourself with sunburn. The sooner you can soothe the burn, protect and hydrate the damaged skin, and restore normal color, the healthier your skin will remain for the long term.

NEAT TREATMENT

3 drops tea tree essential oil

1. Using your fingertips, apply the undiluted tea tree oil to the burned areas.
2. Repeat this treatment 2 or 3 times a day until the skin is no longer red and painful.

SPRAY

1 ounce purified water
½ teaspoon aloe vera carrier oil
2 to 4 drops lavender essential oil
1 drop helichrysum essential oil

1. Pour the water and aloe vera carrier oil into a small glass spray bottle.
2. Add the lavender and helichrysum essential oils to the water, and shake well to blend.
3. Spritz this blend on your skin.
4. Repeat this treatment as needed until the skin is no longer red and painful.[40]

SCREENING OUT THE SUN Skin cancer has become the most common form of cancer in the United States, with diagnoses of more than 3.5 million cases of skin cancer annually—more than the combined incidence of breast, prostate, lung, and colon cancer. Sunburn is the leading cause of melanoma, the deadliest of skin cancers—in fact, if you have been sunburned more than five times in your life, your risk of melanoma doubles.[41] The blends described here have not been tested by regulatory organizations, so there is no hard evidence about their SPF properties, but their ingredients do offer possibilities for natural sun protection.

SIMPLE SUNSCREEN

4 ounces coconut carrier oil
12 drops Roman chamomile essential oil
10 drops lavender essential oil
10 drops helichrysum essential oil
8 drops myrrh essential oil

1. Pour the coconut carrier oil into a small glass or ceramic bowl.
2. Add the Roman chamomile, lavender, helichrysum, and myrrh essential oils to the carrier oils, and stir to combine.
3. Pour the blend into a dark-colored glass bottle that closes tightly, and store the bottle in the refrigerator between uses.
4. Use the blend liberally on exposed skin before going outdoors.
5. Repeat this treatment every 2 to 3 hours for adequate protection.

POWERFUL SUN BLOCK

½ cup sweet almond carrier oil
¼ cup coconut carrier oil
¼ cup beeswax
1 teaspoon red raspberry seed carrier oil
1 teaspoon carrot seed carrier oil
1 teaspoon vitamin E oil
2 tablespoons shea butter
10 drops helichrysum essential oil
10 drops lavender essential oil
2 tablespoons zinc oxide powder

1. Pour the sweet almond and coconut carrier oils into a 16-ounce glass jar.
2. Add the beeswax, red raspberry seed and carrot seed carrier oils, and vitamin E oil, and stir to combine.
3. Add the shea butter to the mixture, and stir to combine.
4. Add the helichrysum and lavender essential oils to the mixture, and stir to combine.
5. Fill a saucepan with several inches of water, and place the saucepan over medium heat.

6. Loosely put the lid on the jar, and place the jar in the pan of heating water to melt the lotion ingredients.
7. As the water heats, stir the ingredients to combine them.
8. When the mixture has melted and is fully combined, add the zinc oxide powder, and stir to combine.
9. Remove the jar from the heat and let the blend cool.
10. Pour the cooled blend into a dark-colored glass jar that closes tightly, and store it in the refrigerator between uses.
11. Use this treatment whenever you go outside; reapply it after swimming or physical activity that causes perspiration.[42]

Tendinitis

Any number of strains, sprains, or repetitive-motion activities can lead to tendinitis, a strain of the fibrous material that links the end of a muscle to the bones of a joint. At worst, a prolonged case of tendinitis can prevent you from working, especially if your job caused the issue.

MASSAGE BLEND

1 ounce olive or sweet almond carrier oil
4 drops helichrysum essential oil
4 drops lemongrass essential oil
2 drops cypress essential oil

1. Pour the olive carrier oil into a small glass or ceramic bowl.
2. Add the helichrysum, lemongrass, and cypress essential oils to the carrier oil, and stir to combine.
3. Pour the blend into a dark-colored glass bottle that closes tightly, and store the bottle in the refrigerator between uses.
4. Using your fingertips, apply the blend into the injured area, and massage it into the skin.
5. Repeat this treatment 2 times a day until the inflammation and pain subsides.

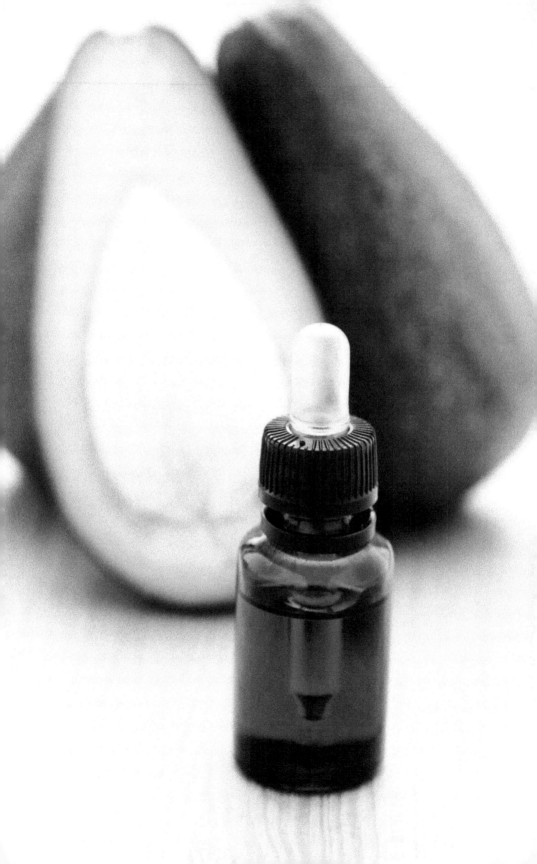

1 ounce avocado carrier oil
10 drops eucalyptus essential oil

1. Pour the avocado carrier oil into a small glass or ceramic bowl.
2. Add the eucalyptus essential oil to the carrier oil, and stir to combine.
3. Pour the blend into a small, dark-colored glass bottle to carry with you.
4. Using your fingertips, apply the blend into the injured area, and massage it into the skin.
5. Repeat this treatment 2 or 3 times a day until the inflammation and pain subsides.

WARM COMPRESS

2 cups warm water
2 drops helichrysum essential oil
2 drops lemongrass essential oil
2 drops peppermint essential oil

1. Follow the instructions in chapter 3 for making a warm compress (page 48).
2. Place the warm compress on the painful area.
3. Remove the compress when it cools to body temperature.
4. Repeat this treatment 3 times a day until the pain subsides and range of motion improves.

Testicle Inflammation

When a testicle is inflamed—a condition known as *orchitis*—pain is usually the most prevalent symptom. There may also be fever, blood in the semen, burning during urination, and a feeling of heaviness in the affected testicle.

1 teaspoon olive carrier oil
2 drops eucalyptus essential oil
2 drops tea tree essential oil
1 drop lavender essential oil

1. Pour the olive carrier oil into a small glass or ceramic bowl.
2. Add the eucalyptus, tea tree, and lavender essential oils to the carrier oil, and stir to combine.
3. Using your fingertips, apply the blend to the affected area, and massage it into the skin.
4. Repeat this treatment 2 times a day until the swelling subsides.

1 teaspoon olive carrier oil
2 drops hyssop essential oil
1 drop Roman chamomile essential oil

1. Pour the olive carrier oil into a small glass or ceramic bowl.
2. Add the hyssop and Roman chamomile essential oils to the carrier oil, and stir to combine.
3. Using your fingertips, apply the blend to the affected area over the Swelling-Reduction Blend in this section, and massage it into the skin.
4. Repeat this treatment 2 times a day until the swelling subsides.

WHEN TO SEE A DOCTOR Most cases of orchitis require antibiotics to be cured completely. See your doctor right away if you have a high fever along with the swelling, if your urination is painful, or if you are an adult with the mumps.

Tick Bite

If you live in an area where deer ticks carry Lyme disease, you know that finding a tick on your body is no joke. Lyme disease becomes a chronic illness with debilitating symptoms, including fatigue, depression, headache, fever, and a circular skin rash. If it's left untreated, it can travel to the central nervous system, your joints, and even your heart. Early treatment can eliminate the symptoms entirely.

NEAT TRICK FOR A TICK

1 drop oregano essential oil

1. Using your fingertip or a cotton swab, apply the undiluted oregano essential oil directly to the tick. You'll need the full strength to kill it, so don't dilute it even though it will burn your skin a little.
2. When the tick loosens its hold, use fine-tipped tweezers to grasp it as close to the skin's surface as possible. Pull it straight up out of your skin. Do not twist it, since this may break off the mouth and leave it lodged in your skin.
3. Save the tick in a small plastic bag to take to your doctor.

NEAT BLEND

2 drops citronella essential oil
2 drops lavender essential oil
2 drops lemongrass essential oil
2 drops rosemary essential oil
2 drops tea tree essential oil

1. Transfer the citronella, lavender, lemongrass, rosemary, and tea tree essential oils to a small, dark-colored glass bottle that closes tightly, and store the bottle in the refrigerator between uses.
2. Using your fingertip, apply 1 drop of the undiluted blend to the site of the wound.
3. If these neat oils sting and burn, apply 1 drop of tea tree essential oil over the antibacterial blend to soothe the burning. Tea tree also provides extra antiseptic properties to help nip the disease in the bud.
4. Repeat this treatment 3 times a day until the bite heals.[43]

WHEN TO SEE A DOCTOR If you begin to experience symptoms of Lyme disease, seek immediate medical attention to eradicate the disease before it spreads through your system.

Tinnitus

Ringing, buzzing, clicking, or random cricket-like sounds in the ears is known as tinnitus, and the symptoms can be so mild that you hardly notice them or so disruptive that you can't sleep. Older adults experience tinnitus more frequently as a reaction to a medication, a side effect of hearing loss, or a symptom of another chronic health problem.

NEAT BLEND

2 drops basil essential oil
2 drops frankincense essential oil

1. Place 1 drop each of undiluted frankincense and basil essential oils on the tip of your index finger.
2. Apply the drops to the back of the ear, and run your finger down your jaw line to your chin.
3. Place the remaining drop each of frankincense and basil essential oils on the tip of your index finger.
4. Apply the drops to the top of the ear, and run your finger down the front of the ear and down the jaw line to your chin.
5. Repeat this treatment every 1 to 4 hours until the ringing stops.

SILENCING BLEND

4 drops cypress essential oil
4 drops helichrysum essential oil
4 drops lavender essential oil
4 drops rosemary essential oil
1 ounce coconut carrier oil

1. Transfer the cypress, helichrysum, lavender, and rosemary essential oils in a small, dark-colored glass bottle, and shake well to blend.
2. Let the essential oil blend stand for 24 hours.
3. Add 1 ounce of coconut carrier oil to the essential oils, and shake well to blend.

4. Put 5 drops of this blend in your palm.
5. Using your fingertip, apply the blend to the front of the ear, around the outside rim of the ear to the lobe, and behind and below the ear, continuing down the jaw line.
6. Repeat the application on the affected ear(s) until you've used up the 5 drops in your palm.
7. Repeat this treatment 2 or 3 times a day until the ringing stops.[44]

Toenail Fungus

Black fungus growing on a thickened toenail can be very difficult to treat effectively, but essential oils that have antifungal properties offer an inexpensive way to deal with this condition.

ANTIFUNGAL BLEND

1 tablespoon jojoba carrier oil
3 drops lavender essential oil
3 drops rosemary essential oil
3 drops tea tree essential oil

1. Pour the jojoba carrier oil into a small glass or ceramic bowl.
2. Add the lavender, rosemary, and tea tree essential oils to the carrier oil, and stir to combine.
3. Using a cotton ball (or several, if more than one toenail is being treated), apply this blend to the affected nail(s) and hold it in place for 10 minutes.
4. Repeat this treatment 3 or 4 times a day until the fungus clears up.

SOAK

Warm water
1 cup apple cider vinegar
10 drops lavender essential oil
10 drops rosemary essential oil
10 drops tea tree essential oil

1. Pour enough warm water to cover your ankles into a glass or ceramic bowl or basin.
2. Add the apple cider vinegar along with the lavender, rosemary, and tea tree essential oils to the water.
3. Put your feet in the water and soak for 20 to 30 minutes.
4. Repeat this treatment at least 2 times a day until the fungus clears up.

Urinary Tract Infection

Also known as *cystitis,* a urinary tract infection (UTI) is an inflammation of the bladder caused by bacteria. UTIs cause a wide range of discomforts, including pain during urination and the constant sensation of needing to urinate. One treatment that couldn't hurt and may actually help is to increase your urine output by drinking all the chamomile tea you can stand, made from dried chamomile in teabags.

WHEN TO SEE A DOCTOR If you see blood or pus in your urine or are running a high fever, you need medical attention, because a UTI can cause even more widespread infections. In an elderly person, a UTI often causes no overt physical symptoms at all, but a UTI can be suspected if there is a sudden onset of psychological symptoms like hallucinations and paranoia.

ANTIBACTERIAL BLEND

1 cup water
30 drops bergamot essential oil

1. Pour the water into a glass measuring cup.
2. Add the bergamot essential oil to the water, and bring it to a boil in your microwave oven.
3. Boil the blend for 1 minute, then let it cool to body temperature.
4. Using a clean cotton ball, swab the urethra area with the blend.
5. Store the unused water in a glass bottle at room temperature.
6. Repeat this treatment 3 times a day until the symptoms of the UTI subside.

Varicose Veins

Long lines and clusters of red, blue, or purple vein lines on your legs are varicose veins—another name for broken blood vessels. When the vessel breaks, the blood pools in your leg, pressing on the vein walls and making them larger. The veins become weaker and start to twist, and you see them as varicose veins. They do not have to be permanent.

MOISTURIZING BLEND

3 drops bergamot essential oil
3 drops ylang-ylang essential oil
6 drops olive carrier oil

1. Place the drops of bergamot and ylang-ylang essential oils in the palm of your hand.
2. Add the olive carrier oil to the essential oils, and rub your palms together 3 times in a circular motion to blend the oils.
3. Apply the blend onto the affected area, starting below the veins and moving upward toward your heart, smoothing it into the skin for about 2 minutes.
4. Repeat this treatment 2 or 3 times a day until the varicose veins fade (about 2 to 3 weeks).

COLD PACK

1 pint refrigerated water
10 drops German chamomile, helichrysum, or rose essential oil

1. Pour the water into a glass or ceramic bowl or low basin.
2. Add the German chamomile essential oil to the water.
3. Follow the instructions in chapter 3 for making a cold pack (page 46).
4. Keep the cold pack in place for 15 to 20 minutes, replacing the water with freshly refrigerated water as necessary.
5. Repeat this treatment 2 or 3 times a day until the varicose veins fade.

....

1 ounce olive, sunflower, or sweet almond carrier oil
25 drops cypress essential oil

1. Pour the olive carrier oil into a small glass or ceramic bowl.
2. Add the cypress essential oil to the carrier oil, and stir to combine.
3. Using your fingertips, apply this blend to the affected area above the varicose veins, and massage it into the skin. (Avoid massaging below the blood vessel—that puts more pressure on the capillary and can prolong the healing process.)
4. Repeat this treatment 2 or 3 times a day until the varicose veins fade.

Warts

Warts seem like the stuff of fairy tales until one appears on your hand, foot, or face. Warts come from the human papilloma virus (HPV), and they can appear on any human being. To eradicate one in short order, use an antiviral essential oil applied directly to the site.

NEAT ANTIVIRAL BLEND
....

1 drop cypress essential oil
1 drop lemon essential oil

Apply 1 drop of each undiluted essential oil on the wart 2 times a day until the wart shrinks.

SAFETY REMINDER Be sure to keep the wart out of the sun, since lemon oil is photosensitive and could form a spot where the wart was.

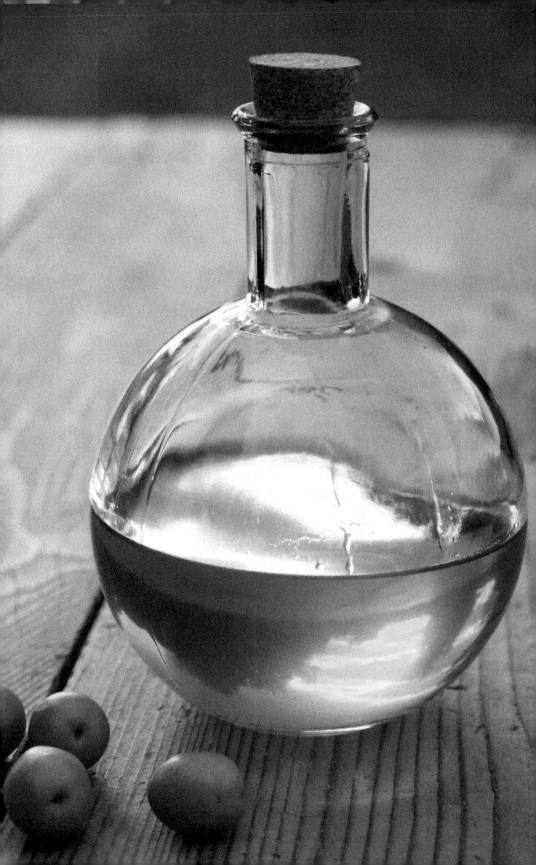

Wasp Sting

While bee and hornet stings are very similar in chemical nature, wasp stings are different—they are alkaline and require specific treatment.

DAB-ON TREATMENT

1 teaspoon vinegar
2 drops lavender or chamomile essential oil

1. Pour the vinegar into a small glass or ceramic bowl.
2. Add the lavender essential oil to the vinegar, and stir to combine.
3. Using a cotton ball, dab the blend onto the sting.
4. Repeat this treatment 3 times a day until the pain and swelling subside.

NEAT TREATMENT

1 drop basil, German chamomile, or lavender essential oil

Using your fingertip, apply the undiluted basil essential oil directly to the sting to help reduce pain and swelling.

Water Retention

Uncomfortable fluid retention can cause swelling in your feet, ankles, hands, wrists, or legs. This often comes from sitting in one place or position for a long time, a diet high in salt, or you have an illness that causes edema.

MASSAGE BLEND

10 drops cypress essential oil
10 drops fennel essential oil
10 drops geranium essential oil
10 drops grapefruit essential oil
10 drops juniper berry essential oil
½ ounce calendula or sunflower carrier oil

1. Transfer the cypress, fennel, geranium, grapefruit, and juniper berry essential oils into a small, dark-colored glass bottle, and shake to combine.
2. Add 6 drops of this blend to the calendula carrier oil in a small glass or ceramic bowl, and stir to combine.
3. Using your fingertips, apply the blend to the area of fluid retention, massaging in strokes that lead up or in toward the heart.
4. Repeat this treatment 2 or 3 times a day as needed until the swelling from fluid retention subsides.

SOAK

Warm water
10 drops cypress essential oil
10 drops fennel essential oil
10 drops geranium essential oil
10 drops grapefruit essential oil
10 drops juniper berry essential oil

1. Pour enough warm water to cover your ankles into a glass or ceramic bowl or basin.
2. Transfer the cypress, fennel, geranium, grapefruit, and juniper berry essential oils into a small, dark-colored glass bottle, and shake to combine.
3. Put 3 to 8 drops of the essential oil blend into the water.
4. Put your feet in the water and soak for 10 to 15 minutes.[45]

Whooping Cough

The familiar whooping sound a child makes when he has this bacterial infection strikes fear in the heart of any parent. The coughing comes in fits that make the child gasp for air. Modern medicine has proven cures for this infection and your child should have the fastest, safest, and most effective medicine available to you. Essential oils should be used only as complementary remedies.

2 ounces sweet almond carrier oil
20 drops eucalyptus essential oil
5 drops basil essential oil
5 drops cedarwood essential oil
5 drops peppermint essential oil

1. Pour the sweet almond carrier oil into a small glass or ceramic bowl.
2. Add the eucalyptus, basil, cedarwood, and peppermint essential oils to the carrier oil, and stir to combine.
3. Rub the blend on the child's chest.
4. Repeat this treatment 2 or 3 times a day to loosen congestion until the infection passes.

WARNING: NOT FOR INFANTS AND TODDLERS Do not use this rub with children younger than two years old, since the eucalyptus and peppermint oils can cause a spasm in the throat muscles, closing off the airway.[46]

DIFFUSER BLEND
....

20 drops eucalyptus essential oil
20 drops lavender essential oil

1. Combine the eucalyptus and lavender essential oils in a small, dark-colored glass bottle, and shake well to blend.
2. Add 3 drops of the blend to a diffuser, and run it in your child's room for 10 to 15 minutes every 3 hours until the congestion passes.

Notes

1. I. B. Bassett, D. L. Pannowitz, and R. S. Barnetson, "A Comparative Study of Tea-Tree Oil versus Benzoylperoxide in the Treatment of Acne," *Medical Journal of Australia* 153:8 (1990), 455–58, http://www.ncbi.nlm.nih.gov/pubmed/2145499; see also S. Enshaieh, A. Jooya, A. H. Siadat, and F. Iraji, "The Efficacy of 5% Topical Tea Tree Oil Gel in Mild to Moderate Acne Vulgaris: A Randomized, Double-Blind, Placebo-Controlled Study," *Indian Journal of Dermatology, Venereology and Leprology* 73:1 (2007), 22–25, http://www.ncbi.nlm.nih.gov/pubmed/17314442.

2. Valerie Ann Worwood, *The Complete Book of Essential Oils and Aromatherapy: Over 600 Natural, Nontoxic, and Fragrant Recipes to Create Health, Beauty, a Safe Home Environment* (Novato, CA: New World Library, 1991), chap. 6; see also Valerie Ann Worwood, *The Fragrant Pharmacy: A Complete Guide to Aromatherapy and Essential Oils* (New York: Bantam, 1991).

3. Kathi Keville, "How to Treat Asthma with Aromatherapy," HowStuffWorks, April 25, 2007, health.howstuffworks.com/wellness/natural-medicine/aromatherapy/how-to-treat-asthma-with-aromatherapy.htm.

4. Matt Jabs, "Simple and Effective Homemade Deodorant," DIY Natural, accessed July 8, 2014, www.diynatural.com/natural-homemade-deodorant.

5. "Bruises," Oils and Plants, accessed July 8, 2014, www.oilsandplants.com/bruises.htm.

6. Ibid.

7. Ray Miller, "Bunions," Sharing the Health, accessed July 8, 2014, http://sharingthehealth .com/index.php/health-concerns/92-bunions.

8. "Summary of the Evidence for Aromatherapy and Essential Oils," National Cancer Institute at the National Institutes of Health, accessed July 6, 2014, http://www.cancer. gov/cancertopics/pdq/cam/aromatherapy/healthprofessional/; see also T. K. Lai, M. C. Cheung, C. K. Lo, K. L. Ng, Y. H. Fung, M. Tong, and C. C. Yau, "Effectiveness of Aroma Massage on Advanced Cancer Patients with Constipation: A Pilot Study," *Complementary Therapies in Clinical Practice* 17:1 (2011), 37–43, http://www.ncbi.nlm.nih.gov /pubmed/21168113?dopt=Abstract.

9. Amy Austin, "Chicken Pox and Essential Oils," *Healthy Families with Only Naturals* (blog), January 27, 2014, http://onlynaturals.wordpress.com/2014/01/27 /chicken-pox-and-essential-oils.

10. Ibid.

11. Lindsey Z, "Natural Cures for Keratosis Pilaris," *The Accidental Wallflower* (blog), July 23, 2013, www.theaccidentalwallflower.com/2013/07/natural-cures-for-keratosis -pilaris.html.

12. Worwood, *Complete Book of Essential Oils and Aromatherapy*.

13. Penny Keay, "Are There Essential Oils That Can Help Cold Sores & Fever Blisters?," Birch Hill Happenings Aromatherapy, accessed July 10, 2014, birchhillhappenings.com /aromatip/1192011coldsores.pdf.

14. Worwood, *Complete Book of Essential Oils and Aromatherapy*.

15. Amanda Herron, "What Essential Oils to Use for Cracked Heels," LiveStrong, last updated January 28, 2014, www.livestrong.com/article/136456-what-essential-oils -use-cracked-heels.

16. Worwood, *Complete Book of Essential Oils and Aromatherapy*.

17. Mohamed Fawzy Ramadan, Mohamed Mostafa Afify Amer, and Ahmed El-Said Awad, "Coriander (*Coriandrum sativum L.*) Seed Oil Improves Plasma Lipid Profile in Rats Fed a Diet Containing Cholesterol," *European Food Research and Technology* 227:4 (2008), 1173–82, www.researchgate.net/publication/225346029_Coriander_(Coriandrum _sativum_L.)_seed_oil_improves_plasma_lipid_profile_in_rats_fed_a_diet_containing _cholesterol; see also Tina Sartorius, Andreas Peter, Nadja Schulz, Andrea Drescher, Ina Bergheim, Jürgen Machann, Fritz Schick, et al., "Cinnamon Extract Improves Insulin

Sensitivity in the Brain and Lowers Liver Fat in Mouse Models of Obesity," *PLoS One* 9:3 (2014), e92358, www.ncbi.nlm.nih.gov/pmc/articles/PMC3958529.

18. Worwood, *Complete Book of Essential Oils and Aromatherapy*.

19. Shellie Enteen, "Essential Oils for Fibromyalgia," *Massage Today* 6:3 (2006), www .massagetoday.com/mpacms/mt/article.php?id=13377.

20. Ibid.

21. Tieraona Low Dog, "3 Best Essential Oils for Cold and Flu," *Prevention*, September 2013, www.prevention.com/health/health-concerns/best-essential-oils-cold-and-flu.

22. Katie, "Luxurious Homemade Lotion Recipe," *Wellness Mama* (blog), accessed July 11, 2014, wellnessmama.com/3765/luxurious-homemade-lotion-recipe.

23. H. Göbel, G. Schmidt, and D. Soyka, "Effect of Peppermint and Eucalyptus Oil Preparations on Neurophysiological and Experimental Algesimetric Headache Parameters," *Cephalagia* 14:3 (1994), 228–34, www.ncbi.nlm.nih.gov/pubmed/7954745.

24. "Which Essential Oils Can Be Used to Treat Hives?," Curiosity, accessed July 12, 2014, curiosity.discovery.com/question/get-rid-of-hives-with.

25. Kathi Keville, "Treating Insect Bites with Aromatherapy," HowStuffWorks, May 1, 2007, health.howstuffworks.com/wellness/natural-medicine/aromatherapy/treating -insect-bites-with-aromatherapy.htm.

26. Ibid.

27. Danny Kingsley, "Catnips Sends Mozzies Flying," ABC, September 3, 2001, www.abc .net.au/science/news/health/HealthRepublish_355524.htm.

28. Jeff Callahan, "Top 10 Essential Oils for Sleep & Insomnia," EssentialOilBenefits.org, May 10, 2013, http://essentialoilbenefits.org/top-10-essential-oils-sleep-insomnia.

29. Tieraona Low Dog, "3 Ways to Cool Hot Flashes," *Prevention*, July 2013, www.prevention.com/health/health-concerns/natural-remedies-hot-flashes.

30. M. H. Hur, M. S. Lee, K. Y. Seong, and M. K. Lee, "Aromatherapy Massage on the Abdomen for Alleviating Menstrual Pain in High School Girls: A Preliminary Controlled Clinical Study," *Evidence-Based Complementary and Alternative Medicine*, 2012, accessed July 13, 2014, www.ncbi.nlm.nih.gov/pubmed/21949670.

31. Aksel Grøntved, Torben Brask, Jørgen Kambskard, and Erwin Hentzer, "Ginger Root Against Seasickness: A Controlled Trial on the Open Sea," *Acta Oto-laryngologica* 105:1–2 (1988), 45–49, http://informahealthcare.com/doi/abs/10.3109/00016488809119444; see also J. J. Stewart, M. J. Wood, C. D. Wood, and M. E. Mims, "Effects of Ginger on Motion Sickness Susceptibility and Gastric Function," *Pharmacology* 42:2 (1991), 111–20, www .ncbi.nlm.nih.gov/pubmed/2062873.

32. Lea Harris, "Essential Oils 101: Using Essential Oils for Muscle-Related Pain Relief," Nourishing Treasures, March 8, 2013, http://www.nourishingtreasures.com/index .php/2013/03/08/essential-oils-101-using-essential-oils-for-muscle-related-pain-relief.

33. "Nose Bleed," Esoteric Oils, accessed July 14, 2014, www.essentialoils.co.za/treatment /nose-bleed.htm.

34. R. C. Mühlbauer, A. Lozano, S. Palacio, A. Reinli, and R. Felix, "Common Herbs, Essential Oils, and Monoterpenes Potently Modulate Bone Metabolism," *Bone* 32:4 (2003), 372–80, http://www.ncbi.nlm.nih.gov/pubmed/12689680.

35. Elizabeth Shogren, "Why Dawn Is the Bird Cleaner of Choice in Oil Spills," *Morning Edition*, June 22, 2010, http://www.npr.org/templates/story/story .php?storyId=127999735.

36. Kathi Keville, "Aromatherapy Sore Throat Cure," HowStuffWorks, May 1, 2007, http://health.howstuffworks.com/wellness/natural-medicine/aromatherapy /aromatherapy-sore-throat-cure.htm.

37. Kathi Keville, "Aromatherapy Stress Relief," HowStuffWorks, May 1, 2007, http:// health.howstuffworks.com/wellness/natural-medicine/aromatherapy/aromatherapy -stress-relief.htm.

38. Worwood, *Complete Book of Essential Oils and Aromatherapy*.

39. Victoria H. Edwards, *The Aromatherapy Companion: Medicinal Uses, Ayurvedic Healing, Body-Care Blends, Perfumes and Scents, Emotional Health and Well-Being* (North Adams, MA: Storey Publishing, 1999), 231.

40. "Home Remedies for Sunburn Provide Cooling Relief with Essential Oils," Experience-Essential-Oils, accessed June 25, 2014, www.experience-essential-oils.com /home-remedies-for-sunburn.html.

41. "Skin Cancer Facts," Skin Cancer Foundation, last modified June 4, 2014, www .skincancer.org/skin-cancer-information/skin-cancer-facts#general.

42. Katie, "Natural Homemade Sunscreen," *Wellness Mama* (blog), accessed June 25, 2014, http://wellnessmama.com/2558/homemade-sunscreen.

43. Jo Pedranti, "Essential Oils and Ticks," *Jo's Health Corner* (blog), accessed June 25, 2014, http://joshealthcorner.blogspot.com/2013/04/essential-oils-ticks.html.

44. "Tinnitus," EverythingEssential, accessed June 25, 2014, http://www .everythingessential.me/HealthConcerns/Tinnitus.html#page=page-2.

45. "Essential Oils and Fluid Retention," West Coast Institute of Aromatherapy, accessed June 22, 2014, www.westcoastaromatherapy.com/free-information/articles-archive /essential-oils-and-fluid-retention.

46. Penny Keay, "Whooping Cough (Pertussis): Using Essential Oils to Help," Birch Hill Happenings Aromatherapy, accessed June 25, 2014, http://birchhillhappenings.com /v1592012whoopingcough.htm.

5

WELLNESS AND BEAUTY BOOSTS

Essential oils can bring
about noticeable improvements
in the way you look

Aromatherapy can support your health and well-being, but its most pleasing effects come to light when you use it for hair, facial, skin, nail, and overall body care. Essential oils don't just smell good. They can also bring about noticeable improvements in the way you look. Making your own creams, lotions, balms, and other personal care items is one sure way to know the products you're using contain only natural ingredients, including pure essential oils.

If you don't already have a natural foods store at which you shop, look for one in your area. You'll find ingredients like castile soap, rosewater, raw cocoa butter, raw honey, and vegetable glycerin at your neighborhood co-op grocery story, public market, or natural foods store (in larger cities, try Whole Foods or Trader Joe's).

It may surprise you to find how easy it is to mix your own beauty products—and once you begin using these natural ingredients, you may find it more economical than buying expensive department store products loaded with chemicals you can't pronounce. Perhaps best of all, you can customize the scents of your homemade bath balls, bath salts, deodorant, lip balm, and lip gloss to suit your senses, selecting just the right balance of scents from the suggested lists in these recipes, or from the apothecary in chapter 8.

Astringent

For oily, combination, or acne-prone skin, use essential oils with an astringent effect. Place a few drops of this astringent onto a cotton ball and smooth it over your face, paying special attention to the T-zone area.

2 ounces rosewater
1 ounce witch hazel
2 drops sandalwood essential oil
1 drop cypress essential oil

1. Pour the rosewater into a 3-ounce glass bottle.
2. Add the witch hazel, followed by the sandalwood and cypress essential oils, and shake well.
3. Let the solution stand for 36 hours.
4. Shake the solution again, and pour it through a coffee filter to remove the oils sitting on top of the mixture.
5. Discard the filter, and pour the remaining solution back into the bottle.

Bath Balls

Toss two of these in the bathwater to delight your children or give yourself a treat. A basket or bowl of these fragrant little wonders also makes a nice addition to a bathroom shelf or vanity.

½ cup citric acid
1 cup baking soda
¾ cup cornstarch
¼ cup Epsom salt
10 to 15 drops essential oil (good choices: jasmine, lavender, patchouli, vanilla, and ylang-ylang)
6 drops food coloring of your choice
2 ounces water

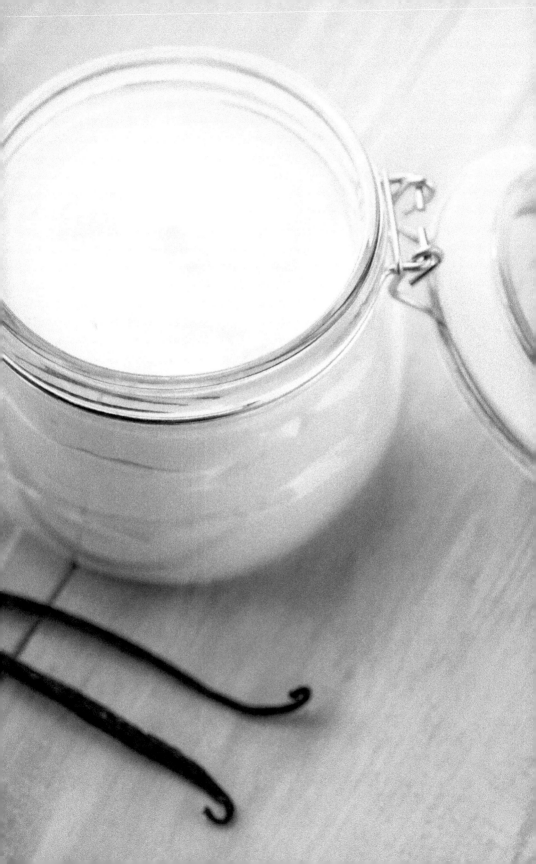

1. Stir together the citric acid, baking soda, and cornstarch, and run them through a sifter or sieve to be sure they're thoroughly combined.
2. Add the Epsom salt, and mix thoroughly.
3. Add the essential oil and food coloring to the dry ingredients, using your fingers to break up any lumps.
4. Lightly spray the mixture with the water to dampen it. If you use too much water, the mixture will fizz and expand.
5. Form the dampened mixture into round balls about the size of an egg.
6. Place the balls on a baking sheet, and leave them to dry overnight.
7. Store the bath balls where they'll be within easy reach for a soothing bath.[1]

Bath Salts

It takes only a few minutes to create your own bath salts, and you can store them in attractive containers for display on your bathroom shelves.

3 cups sea salt
3 teaspoons coconut carrier oil
6 drops cedarwood essential oil
6 drops chamomile essential oil
4 drops clary sage essential oil
4 drops jasmine essential oil

1. Pour the salt into a ceramic or glass bowl.
2. Drizzle the coconut carrier oil over the salt 1 teaspoon at a time, mixing after each drizzle to prevent clumping.

3. Add the cedarwood, chamomile, clary sage, and jasmine essential oils, and mix well.
4. Store the salts in a container with a tight-fitting lid, and add up to 1 cup to a running bath.

MAKE A LABEL Several types of "designer drugs" (hallucinogens and powerful synthetic stimulants) are made to resemble legal products and sold under the name *bath salts*. If your bath salts are going to be a gift, reassure the recipient by listing the ingredients on the jar.

Body Butter

It's quick and easy to whip up your own full-body moisturizing butter. If the combined scents of vanilla, almond, coconut, and cocoa sound too sweet, replace the cocoa butter with shea butter, and use jasmine or ylang-ylang essential oil. This recipe yields about 3 cups.

1 cup raw cocoa butter
½ cup coconut carrier oil
½ cup sweet almond carrier oil
6 drops vanilla essential oil

1. Place the cocoa butter and the coconut carrier oil in a glass or ceramic bowl.
2. Set the bowl in a pan of water over low heat, and allow the ingredients to melt.
3. Remove the bowl from the heat and let it cool for 30 minutes.
4. Add the sweet almond carrier oil and the vanilla essential oil to the cooled mixture.
5. Chill the mixture in the freezer for 20 minutes.
6. Using an electric mixer or a food processor, whip the combined ingredients until they look like butter.
7. Spoon the body butter into a glass jar, and store it in the refrigerator between uses.

Cuticle Treatment

For the luxurious feeling of a salon treatment without the expense of a manicure, mix up a batch of this softening soak.

¼ cup sweet almond carrier oil
2 teaspoons apricot kernel carrier oil
5 drops geranium essential oil
2 drops rose essential oil

1. Pour the sweet almond and apricot kernel carrier oils, then the geranium and rose essential oils, into a small dark-colored glass bottle, and shake well.
2. Add a few drops of the solution to a bowl of warm water.
3. Soak your hands for 10 minutes.[2]

Deodorant

If you've had it with aluminum-laden commercial deodorants, make your own deodorant stick, and give it exactly the scent you want. Geranium, lavender, lemon, lemongrass, lime, tea tree, and thyme are all natural antibacterial choices.

¼ cup aluminum-free baking soda
¼ cup arrowroot or cornstarch
15 drops essential oil
3 to 5 tablespoons coconut carrier oil

1. Combine the baking soda, arrowroot, and essential oil in a ceramic or glass bowl.
2. Add the coconut carrier oil 1 tablespoon at a time, working it with a pastry blender until the mixture has the consistency of a paste.
3. Press the paste into an empty deodorant container.
4. Place the deodorant in the refrigerator for 1 hour or until the coconut oil solidifies. Store the deodorant in a cool, dry place.

Facial Cleanser

You can use this all-natural cleanser every day to clarify and tone your skin. It's a combination that's potent against acne, too. Look for the liquid castile soap at a natural foods store.

1 cup filtered water
¼ cup liquid castile soap
5 teaspoons jojoba carrier oil
2 tablespoons raw honey
15 drops lemon essential oil
1 tablespoon tea tree essential oil

1. Pour the water into a glass or ceramic bowl.
2. Add the castile soap to the water.
3. Add the jojoba carrier oil and honey, followed by the lemon and tea tree essential oils, and stir gently.
4. Pour the mixture into a dispenser for foaming soap, and shake before use.[3]

Hair Conditioner

This recipe is for normal hair types. If you have oily hair, use birch or sage instead of lavender. For dry hair, use geranium or yarrow instead of lemon.

2 ounces water
2 ounces white vinegar
½ teaspoon vegetable glycerin
3 drops rosemary essential oil
2 drops lavender essential oil
2 drops lemon essential oil

1. In a dark-colored glass bottle, add the water, vinegar, and vegetable glycerin.
2. Add the rosemary, lavender, and lemon essential oils, and shake well.

3. Wash your hair, and rinse it thoroughly.
4. Pour the conditioner on your wet hair and comb it through.
5. Leave the conditioner in for best results, or rinse after 1 minute.

Lip Balm

Forget about petroleum and factory-made waxes. Use beeswax, shea butter, and carrier oils to keep your lips soft and prevent them from cracking. Best of all, you get to choose the scent. This recipe yields enough lip balm to fill 7 tubes (0.15-ounce size). Make sure the tubes have caps.

½ ounce beeswax
2 teaspoons olive or jojoba carrier oil
2 teaspoons coconut carrier oil
1 teaspoon shea or cocoa butter
½ teaspoon pure aloe vera
¼ teaspoon vitamin E oil
5 to 7 drops eucalyptus, peppermint, spearmint, vanilla, or another essential oil

1. Combine the beeswax, olive and coconut carrier oils, and shea butter in a ceramic or glass bowl.
2. Bring a saucepan of water just to the boiling point, and turn the heat down to a simmer.
3. Place the bowl in the simmering water, and stir the mixture until it melts.
4. Remove the bowl from the heat and stir in the aloe vera, vitamin E oil, and eucalyptus essential oil.
5. Pour the mixture into 0.15-ounce tubes and allow it to cool completely.[4]

Lip Gloss (Clear)

The addition of lanolin, the natural lubricant found in sheep's wool, provides a layer of protection for your lips and a glistening finish to your lipstick. This recipe yields enough gloss to fill 4 half-ounce tins. Make sure the tins have lids.

½ ounce pure beeswax
1 tablespoon olive or jojoba carrier oil
2 teaspoons coconut carrier oil
1 teaspoon shea butter
½ teaspoon castor oil
½ teaspoon lanolin
½ teaspoon pure aloe vera
¼ teaspoon vitamin E oil
5 to 10 drops peppermint, tea tree, vanilla, or another
      essential oil

1. Combine the beeswax, olive and coconut carrier oils, shea butter, castor oil, and lanolin in a ceramic or glass bowl.
2. Bring a saucepan of water just to the boiling point, and turn the heat down to a simmer.
3. Place the bowl in the simmering water, and watch carefully until the beeswax and oils have melted.
4. Remove the bowl from the heat and stir in the aloe vera, vitamin E oil, and peppermint essential oil.
5. Pour the mixture into tins and allow the gloss to cool before securing the lids.[5]

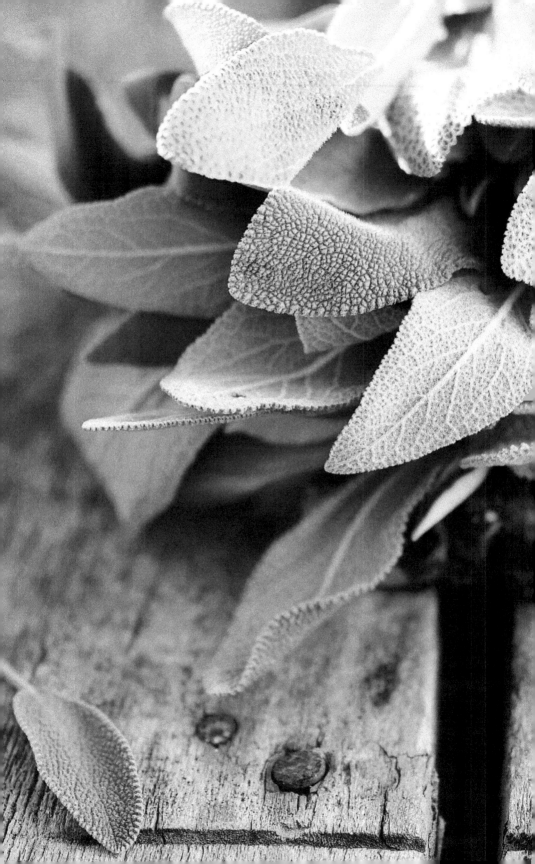

Mask

For oily skin, there's nothing like a facial mask to dissolve the excess and remove dead skin cells. For dry skin, substitute with 10 drops of sandalwood, 5 drops of rose, and 3 drops of patchouli essential oils. If your skin is neither oily nor dry, use 10 drops of lavender, 5 drops of chamomile, and 3 drops of lemon essential oils. Always remember to stay out of the sun for at least 12 hours after using photosensitizing oils (see chapter 8).

3 tablespoons white cornmeal
3 tablespoons freshly ground raw almonds
10 drops lavender essential oil
5 drops bergamot essential oil
3 drops clary sage essential oil
2 to 3 tablespoons water

1. In a glass or ceramic bowl, mix the cornmeal and ground almonds with the lavender, bergamot, and clary sage essential oils.
2. Add the water 1 tablespoon at a time to form a paste.
3. Apply the mask directly to your face, using a circular motion to buff away dead skin cells.
4. Allow the mask to dry and tighten (about 10 minutes).
5. Rinse your face with lukewarm water.[6]

Moisturizer

Wake up dry or aging skin with this rich concoction.

½ ounce beeswax
4 ounces sweet almond carrier oil
21 drops geranium essential oil
12 drops patchouli essential oil
6 drops rose otto essential oil
3 ounces water

1. Combine the beeswax and sweet almond carrier oil in a ceramic or glass bowl.
2. Bring a saucepan of water just to the boiling point, and turn the heat down to a simmer.
3. Place the bowl in the simmering water and watch carefully until the beeswax and oil have melted.
4. Remove the bowl from the heat and let it cool to room temperature.
5. Add the geranium, patchouli, and rose otto essential oils to the cooled mixture.
6. Pour the water into a blender equipped with a lid that has an opening.
7. With the blender set to high, slowly add the mixture of wax and oil in a steady stream through the opening in the lid until the contents of the blender form a creamy emulsion.
8. Pour the emulsion into a glass jar, and close the lid tightly.
9. Store the moisturizer in the refrigerator between uses.[7]

Nail Growth Oil

At bedtime, give your nails some overnight encouragement with this nourishing, stimulating rub.

2 drops lavender essential oil
1 drop myrrh essential oil
1 drop peppermint essential oil
1½ tablespoons sweet almond carrier oil

1. Add the lavender, myrrh, and peppermint essential oils to a ceramic or glass bowl. Stir in the sweet almond carrier oil.
2. Pour the blend into a dark-colored glass bottle that closes tightly, and store the bottle in the refrigerator between uses.
3. Using a cotton swab, apply the blend to your nails once a day at bedtime.

Scrub

A good full-body salt scrub will exfoliate your skin and buff it to a silky sheen. Try this easy recipe for a scrub that you can use liberally in the shower. For a less coarse texture, add some fine table salt until you get the desired consistency.

½ cup coarse sea salt
⅓ cup grape seed or jojoba carrier oil
1 tablespoon dried lavender
15 drops lavender essential oil

1. Combine the salt with the grape seed carrier oil in a ceramic or glass bowl.
2. Add the dried lavender and the lavender essential oil, and mix well.
3. Using a washcloth and about 1 ounce of the blend, scrub your skin, then rinse.

HOLD THE SALT If you're familiar with the idiom *to rub salt into a wound*, then you already know what will happen if you use this scrub when you have an open cut or sore anywhere on your body—it will sting like crazy.[8]

Shampoo

What could be more inviting than honey and coconut as natural hair cleansers? Try this shampoo developed by Nina Nelson of *Shalom Mama* blog. A natural foods store will have the liquid castile soap.

½ cup liquid castile soap
¼ cup canned coconut milk
¼ cup honey
2 tablespoons coconut carrier oil
1 tablespoon vitamin E oil
30 drops wild orange essential oil
20 drops lavender essential oil

1. Combine the soap, coconut milk, honey, coconut carrier oil, and vitamin E oil in a ceramic or glass container with a lid.
2. Add the wild orange and lavender essential oils.
3. Close the container, and shake well to mix thoroughly.
4. Use this blend as you would any other shampoo.[9]

Toner

Tighten and refresh your skin after you wash and before you moisturize using this pure combination of rosewater and essential oils. For oily skin, use juniper berry and rose otto essential oils instead of chamomile and geranium oils. Place a few drops of this toner onto a cotton ball and smooth it over your face, paying special attention to the T-zone area.

3 ounces rosewater
1 drop chamomile essential oil
1 drop geranium essential oil

1. Pour the rosewater into a 4-ounce glass bottle.
2. Add the chamomile and geranium essential oils, and shake well.
3. Let the solution stand for 36 hours.
4. Shake the mixture again, and pour the solution through a coffee filter to remove the oils sitting on top of the mixture.
5. Discard the filter, and pour the remaining solution back into the bottle.

Notes

1. "Bath Fizzies," Scentsable Living, May 22, 2012, http://scentsable-living.com /2012/05/22/bath-fizzies.

2. "Natural Nail Care Recipes," NB Community . . . Natural Beauty, accessed June 29, 2014, http://naturalnailcarerecipes.homestead.com/cuticleoils.html.

3. Nadia, "DIY All-Natural Clarifying and Toning Foaming Facewash," *Body Unburdened* (blog), accessed June 29, 2014, http://bodyunburdened.com/diy-all-natural-toning -clarifying-foaming-facewash.

4. Shaina Olmanson, "Homemade Lip Balm and Lip Gloss For Your Valentine," *Food For My Family* (blog), February 7, 2013, foodformyfamily.com/manic-organic /homemade-lip-balm-and-lip-gloss-for-your-valentine.

5. Ibid.

6. "Skin Care, Moisturizing Cream, Face Mask, Mists," Aura Cacia, accessed June 26, 2014, https://www.auracacia.com/auracacia/aclearn/art_skincare.html.

7. "Rose and Geranium Moisturizing Cream," Aura Cacia, accessed June 26, 2014, http:// www.auracacia.com/recipes/rose-and-geranium-moisturizing-cream.

8. "Lavender Salt Scrub Tutorial," *Queenie and the Dew* (blog), April 17, 2012, http://www .queenieandthedew.com/2012/04/lavender-salt-scrub-tutorial.html#.U6xOUhZ7zaY.

9. Nina Nelson, "Homemade Shampoo with Essential Oils," *Shalom Mama* (blog), October 14, 2013, http://shalommama.com/homemade-shampoo.

6

SIMPLE SCENTS AND PLEASURES

Experiencing your favorite scent
can relieve stress, lighten your mood,
and give you an energizing rush

M aking aromatherapy a normal part of your every-day life is not difficult. At a moment's notice you can relieve stress, lighten your mood, give yourself an energizing rush, or immerse yourself in relaxation when you carry your favorite scent in your briefcase, purse, or pocket, or add it to the atmosphere of your home or car.

You'll find just about all of the ingredients and materials for these items at your local hobby and craft store—with the possible exception of orrisroot, an herb used as a fixative in scented products like holiday wreaths and potpourri. Check for orrisroot at your favorite place to buy exotic spices, or order it online.

It's easy and fun to make all of these items, so they can be a great Saturday-afternoon project for your children. The whole family can be involved in making these items as wedding favors or holiday stocking stuffers, and in creating custom labels and cards to go with them. Scented candles, sachets, sprays, and stationery make wonderful gifts, and they're so simple to create that you can turn them into projects for a middle school class, a scout troop, a summer camp, or the neighborhood kids. Best of all, you will make these gifts entirely with natural ingredients—so you can give with good conscience as well as kindness, knowing that your gift will contribute to the recipient's health and wellness.

Candles

Making your own candle is surprisingly fast and easy. Use your microwave oven, a microwave-safe cup, a glass jar, a craft stick, and a wick to create seasonal candles with holiday scents, or make aromatherapy candles for any time of year. Best of all, your candles will be free of the asthma-aggravating particulate matter found in many commercially scented candles.

2 cups soy wax flakes
2 or 3 drops essential oil of your choice (more if you're using a light scent)

1. Place the soy wax flakes in a microwave-safe cup, such as an 8-ounce Pyrex or other heat-resistant measuring cup. Leave room at the top in case the wax expands and rises while being heated.
2. Place the cup of wax flakes in the microwave, and run the appliance in 10-second increments until the wax has completely liquefied.
3. Pour the liquefied wax into the glass jar that will hold the finished candle (the jar should be small enough for the liquefied wax to fill it).
4. Add the essential oil to the wax, and quickly stir the oil in with the craft stick.
5. Place the wick into the center of the wax, and hold it there for a minute or two while the wax cools enough to keep the wick firmly in place.
6. Trim the wick until only 1 inch remains above the level of the wax.
7. Refrigerate the candle for 2 hours.[1]

Pillow Spray

Move from relaxation into restful sleep with a simple spray for misting your pillow, not to mention your sheets and even the air in your bedroom. Use the oils listed here, or choose another one that encourages peace and tranquillity—bergamot, geranium, lemon, vanilla, ylang-ylang, or others that you can read about in chapter 8.

3 ounces water
2 drops chamomile essential oil
2 drops lavender essential oil
1 drop orange essential oil

1. Add the water and chamomile, lavender, and orange essential oils to a glass or metal spray bottle, and shake well.
2. Use the spray to spritz pillows and the area around the bed.

KEEP THE PEACE Avoid spicy or minty fragrances that stimulate energy. Cinnamon, clove, peppermint, and spearmint are not conducive to good sleep.

Potpourri

There was a time when making your own potpourri meant taking to the woods and hunting for fragrant leaves, cones, and flowers. Today you can forage for these items at a craft store and then go home and add the fragrance yourself. The oils suggested here will yield a pleasantly traditional potpourri scent, with frankincense as a fixative that holds the fragrance. You may also choose to experiment with a different blend. If you do, be sure to use another oil with fixative properties—balsam of Peru, benzoin, cedarwood, myrrh, patchouli, sandalwood, or vetiver.[2]

11 drops orange essential oil
8 drops cinnamon essential oil
6 drops ginger essential oil
4 drops frankincense essential oil

1 drop nutmeg essential oil
Dried plant materials from a craft store

1. Mix the orange, cinnamon, ginger, frankincense, and nutmeg essential oils in a small dark-colored glass bottle.
2. Add 5 to 8 drops of the combined oils to the dried plant material, and toss to blend.
3. Use the remaining oil as necessary to refresh the potpourri.

Sachets

A traditional sachet is a small drawstring bag made of cotton, silk, or organdy and filled with a powder produced from finely ground dried flowers or roots. But you don't have to grind your own. You can find mixes of dried flowers and herbs at a craft store, which may also carry the type of little drawstring bags used for wedding favors, or you can look for the spice or bouquet garni bags sold at stores where cooking supplies are found. When you choose your essential oil, make sure it harmonizes with your plant material (for example, if you're using lavender flowers, use lavender oil). The sachet mix described here uses orrisroot as a fixative.

5 drops essential oil
2 teaspoons orrisroot
Mixed dried flowers and herbs

1. Add the essential oil and orrisroot to the dried plant material, and toss to blend.
2. Use the mixture to fill drawstring bags, and draw the strings closed.
3. Tuck the sachets into drawers or closets to give clothes a delicate scent.

Scented Stationery

Now that you know how to make a sachet, use one to scent some paper for your own notes and letters, or for a special gift. Your gift will be even more special if you include the sachet!

Writing paper from a high-end stationery store
Box with a tightly closing lid
1 sachet

1. Place the stationery in the box.
2. Add the sachet, and replace the lid.
3. Put the box away for at least 2 weeks before using the stationery or presenting it as a gift.

Notes

1. "How to Make a Candle with Essential Oils," WikiHow, accessed June 29, 2014, www.wikihow.com/Make-a-Candle-With-Essential-Oils.

2. "Aromatherapy Potpourri Recipes," AromaWeb, accessed June 29, 2014, www.aromaweb.com/recipes/potpourri.asp.

YOUR NATURAL HOME

You have all the cleaning
products you will ever need, and
they're already in your pantry

A re you a prisoner of the many chemicals you use to clean your home? Sometimes it seems like a different product is needed for every single surface—and every product is loaded with ammonia, chlorine bleach, and a long list of other substances you couldn't pronounce even if you could read the tiny print on the labels.

Well, cheer up! You'll be happy to hear that you already have all the cleaning products you could ever need, and they're right on your pantry shelves and in your bathroom cabinets. They're as good as any commercial mix, but without the mysterious synthetics, and with only half the syllables. If you have a little vinegar, some baking soda, a handful of castile soap flakes, a box of borax, and a few essential oils, you can scrub your floors, clean your counters, and wash your clothes just as effectively as you could with store-bought products, and often at a fraction of the price.

In a number of these recipes, you have the option of customizing the cleaner with the essential oils of your choice, selecting scents from a list of antibacterials. If you enjoy the invigorating scents of citrus and evergreen and you immediately associate lemon and pine with cleanliness, for example, you can choose these powerful germ killers as the main ingredients in your all-purpose cleaner. It's no accident that many commercial cleaning products contain these scents—they do indeed fight bacteria and banish odors. If you prefer the kitchen-friendly scents of cinnamon and clove, however, you can add these germ-fighters to your cleaner instead.

So if you're ready to be released from chemical prison, here are some recipes for good, clean living on the outside.

Several of the projects described in this chapter call for an 8-ounce spray bottle, so be sure yours is made of glass or metal—essential oils will eat through plastic.

Air Freshener

A little water and a few drops of some essential oils can help you banish the stale smells that tend to gather in the corners of a house. Many combinations of oils will get the job done. Experiment with cinnamon and pine for an outdoorsy scent, or try the warm bright notes of orange, clove, and sandalwood.

½ to 1 cup water
8 drops eucalyptus essential oil
8 drops lemon essential oil
8 drops tea tree essential oil

1. Add the water and eucalyptus, lemon, and tea tree essential oils to an 8-ounce glass or metal spray bottle, and shake well.
2. Mist this blend around the house wherever it will do the most good.

TEST YOUR FURNITURE As with all air fresheners, if you plan to apply the spray directly to a piece of furniture, spot test the material first to be sure the mixture won't mar or discolor your favorite recliner or ottoman.

All-Purpose Cleaner

For this cleaner, you can use any of the essential oils that are effective at killing different kinds of bacteria. These include cinnamon, clove, eucalyptus, grapefruit, lavender, lemon, lemongrass, oregano, peppermint, pine, rosemary, tea tree, and thyme oils.

½ cup apple cider vinegar
½ cup water
20 drops essential oil

1. Add the apple cider vinegar, water, and essential oil to an 8-ounce glass or metal spray bottle, and shake well.

2. Use this solution to clean and disinfect your home and leave your space smelling fresh.

COVER THE WATERFRONT Different essential oils kill different kinds of bacteria, so it's a good idea to choose a mix of five or six oils. That way, you won't overlook any of the little nasties that may be doing their dirty work in your kitchen or bathroom.

Bathroom Cleaner

Tea tree essential oil is especially effective at killing mold and mildew in bathrooms. To eliminate mildew, you can apply the oil neat to the caulking and grout in and around your bathtub. You can also mix it into a spray. For that, you'll need an 8-ounce glass or metal spray bottle.

2 cups water
2 teaspoons tea tree essential oil

1. Add the water and tea tree essential oil to a glass or metal spray bottle, and shake well.
2. Spritz the solution on mold or mildew without rinsing. Let it go to work on the stains!

Bathtub Cleaner

Here's all you need to get rid of that waxy soap buildup.

1 cup baking soda
24 drops grapefruit essential oil
24 drops tea tree oil

1. In a small bowl, stir together the baking soda and grapefruit and tea tree essential oils.

2. Sprinkle the powder in the bathtub, and scrub it with a sponge or a brush.
3. Rinse and enjoy a clean bathtub.

Dryer Ball

Add a pleasant fragrance to your clothes as they go through the dryer. Sprinkle a dryer ball or a thick paper towel with a few drops of lavender essential oil or another favorite essential oil, and toss the ball or towel in with the drying laundry.

Fabric Softener

Why bother trying to understand all the crazy chemicals in commercial fabric softeners when you can duplicate or surpass their effects with this do-it-yourself concoction?

½ **cup vinegar**
2 tablespoons baking soda
½ **teaspoon lavender essential oil**

1. In a small bowl, add the vinegar and baking soda and let it dissolve.
2. Add the lavender essential oil.
3. Pour the liquid directly into the washing machine (or its fabric-softener compartment) during the rinse cycle.

Floor Cleaner

A treat for the eyes and the nose, too, this refreshing cleaner brightens your floors and gives them an enjoyable scent.

2 tablespoons unscented liquid soap
1 gallon hot water
3 or 4 drops lemon essential oil
3 or 4 drops tea tree essential oil

1. In a large bucket, add the liquid soap to the hot water, followed by the lemon and tea tree essential oils.
2. Use the mixture as you mop.

Furniture Polish

To make this polish, you'll need a funnel and a 4-ounce glass or metal spray bottle.

4 ounces jojoba carrier oil
12 drops lemon essential oil
8 drops sandalwood essential oil
4 drops lemongrass essential oil

1. Use a funnel to pour the jojoba carrier oil into a glass or metal spray bottle.
2. Add the lemon, sandalwood, and lemongrass essential oils, and shake well.
3. Spray the polish directly onto wood furniture, or spray it on a dust cloth and apply it to furniture.
4. Wipe the furniture with a soft cloth to polish it.

Laundry Detergent (Powder)

Here's a recipe for a detergent powder that will handle 72 loads of laundry. For clean, bright clothes that owe nothing to artificial chemicals, use 2 tablespoons per load.

2 cups castile soap flakes from a box, or grated from a solid bar
4 cups baking soda
3 cups washing soda
3 or 4 drops lavender, lemon, or another favorite essential oil

1. Put the castile soap in a large bowl.
2. Add the baking soda, washing soda, and lavender essential oil, and mix thoroughly.
3. Store the powder in a large jar with a lid that seals tightly.

Toilet Cleaner

You'll need a 22-ounce glass or metal spray bottle to dispense this cleaner.

18 ounces water
¼ cup liquid castile soap
4 drops lavender essential oil
4 drops lemon essential oil
4 drops tea tree essential oil

1. Add the water, castile soap, and lavender, lemon, and tea tree essential oils to the glass or metal spray bottle, and shake well.
2. Spray the mixture in the toilet bowl, and scrub it with a brush.
3. Flush to rinse.

Window Cleaner

It's easy to get sparkling, streak-free windows with this simple cleaner and a glass or metal spray bottle that holds 22 to 32 ounces of liquid.

4 tablespoons white vinegar
12 drops lemon essential oil
Water

1. Using a funnel, pour the vinegar into a glass or metal spray bottle.
2. Add the lemon essential oil, and shake well.
3. Add water to fill the bottle, and shake it again.
4. Spray the cleaner liberally on a window, and wipe the window dry with a crumpled newspaper. Repeat for each window.

8

YOUR
PERSONAL
APOTHECARY

Become a well-informed consumer of
powerful, versatile essential oils with
this quick reference guide

W hat essential oils should you have on hand for yourself and your family? This quick reference guide to more than 60 oils will help you assemble a personal apothecary. It tells you what each oil is good for, how to use it, what it goes with if you want to create a blend, and what to watch out for if you're pregnant, planning to spend some time in the sun, or dealing with a particular ailment or medical condition. In short, this guide is all you need to become a well-informed consumer of powerful, versatile essential oils.

This chapter looks specifically at pure, single essential oils, not at the many blended products that are available from just about any essential oil provider. Before you choose any of these blends—many of which are touted by glowing testimonials on the distributors' websites, or by sales representatives with long-winded spiels—be sure that you know exactly which oils are in them. Blends are meant as conveniences to help speed relief to you for an ailment (or several), but they often contain oils you do not require for that purpose. Just as you would not mix up a handful of pills and swallow them without knowing what you were taking, be cautious in using blends that contain ingredients you do not require. And as with all essential oils, check with your doctor before using any product to be sure it will not react with medications you already take. Be an informed consumer and take the safest path to overall wellness.

Allspice *Pimenta dioica*

Also known as *pimento oil, pimenta,* and *Jamaica pepper,* this yellow-brown oil is similar in scent to clove—warm, spicy, and invigorating. It comes from the West Indies and South America, and it's produced from the plant's leaves or fruit through steam distillation.

WHAT IT'S USED FOR

- Cramps
- Depression
- Flatulence
- Indigestion and nausea
- Neuralgia
- Stress
- Tension

HOW IT'S USED

- In a burner or vaporizer
- In a massage oil blend

COMPLEMENTARY OILS

- Geranium
- Ginger
- Lavender
- Orange
- Patchouli
- Ylang-ylang

WHAT TO WATCH OUT FOR

Allspice oil can cause skin irritation and has been known to irritate the mucous membranes, so use it only in low concentrations.

May cause skin irritation

Aniseed *Pimpinella anisum*

This pungent oil, also known as *anise* and *sweet cumin,* smells like licorice and is not related to star anise. It solidifies at low temperatures, so you may need to warm it with your hands to return it to a liquid. Now cultivated in Europe, Africa, and the United States, aniseed is originally from the Middle East and was used in ancient Greece, Rome, and Egypt. It's also used in liqueurs and toothpastes, and is a breath freshener in India. The oil is produced from the plant's seeds and dried fruit through steam distillation.

WHAT IT'S USED FOR

- Arthritis
- Bronchitis
- Catarrh
- Colic
- Cramps
- Flatulence
- Hangover
- Indigestion
- Migraine and other types of headaches
- Muscle pain
- Stress
- Tension
- Vertigo
- Whooping cough

HOW IT'S USED

- As a neat (undiluted) application on a handkerchief
- In a vaporizer or diffuser

COMPLEMENTARY OILS

- Caraway
- Cardamom
- Cedarwood
- Coriander
- Dill
- Fennel
- Petitgrain
- Rosewood
- Tangerine/mandarin

WHAT TO WATCH OUT FOR

Pregnant women should avoid aniseed oil. The anethole in aniseed oil can cause dermatitis, so aniseed oil should not be used on the skin. Use aniseed oil sparingly—too much can slow circulation and cause cerebral congestion.

Do not use during pregnancy

Do not use on skin

Basil   *Ocimum basilicum*

A light, peppery oil with clear green notes, basil is cultivated throughout Europe and the United States and is a well-known herb in many cuisines. It originated in southern Asia and the Pacific islands, and it's considered sacred to Krishna and Vishnu, two Hindu deities. Basil oil is produced from the plant's leaves and flowers through steam distillation.

WHAT IT'S USED FOR

- Acne
- Allergies
- Arthritis
- Asthma
- Bronchitis
- Constipation
- Gout
- Insect bites
- Menstrual issues
- Migraine and other types of headaches
- Nausea and vomiting
- Nervous disorders

HOW IT'S USED

- In a bath
- In a vaporizer

COMPLEMENTARY OILS

- Bergamot
- Black pepper
- Caraway
- Cedarwood
- Clove
- Fennel
- Geranium
- Ginger
- Grapefruit
- Lavender
- Lemon
- Lemongrass
- Marjoram
- Melissa
- Neroli
- Rose geranium
- Spearmint
- Verbena

Too much basil oil can have a stupefying effect. It should not be used with children younger than 16. Because it can stimulate menstrual flow, pregnant women should avoid basil oil. Basil oil can also irritate the skin.

Do not use during pregnancy

May act as a sedative

May cause skin irritation

Not safe for children under 16

Bay *Laurus nobilis*

Also known as *sweet bay, Mediterranean bay,* and *laurel,* this oil has a spicy-sweet scent. Its source plant is native to the West Indies, Venezuela, and the Guianas, but most of it today comes from Morocco and Spain. Bay was popular with the ancient Romans, who presented Olympic champions with laurel (bay) wreaths to symbolize wisdom and protection. The oil is produced from the plant's leaves through steam distillation.

WHAT IT'S USED FOR

- Arthritis
- Circulatory issues
- Colds and flu
- Diarrhea
- Hair loss or thinning hair
- Neuralgia
- Muscle pain
- Skin infections

HOW IT'S USED

- In a vaporizer or diffuser
- In a massage oil blend
- In a bath

- Cedarwood
- Coriander
- Eucalyptus
- Geranium
- Ginger
- Lavender
- Lemon
- Orange
- Rose
- Rosemary
- Thyme
- Ylang-ylang

WHAT TO WATCH OUT FOR

Be careful about using bay oil on your skin, since it can be irritating. Pregnant women should avoid bay oil.

Do not use during pregnancy

May cause skin irritation

Benzoin *Styrax benzoin*

This resinous oil goes by many other names—*gum benzoin, luban jawi,* and *Benjamin,* for example. With a sweet aroma that recalls vanilla, benzoin has long been an ingredient in incense. The oil is extracted from the resin of a tree that grows in Thailand and on the Indonesian islands of Java and Sumatra.

WHAT IT'S USED FOR

- Acne
- Arthritis
- Bronchitis
- Chilblains
- Circulatory issues
- Colds and coughs
- Depression
- Eczema
- Muscle pain
- Psoriasis
- Rashes
- Scar tissue
- Stress
- Tension
- Wounds

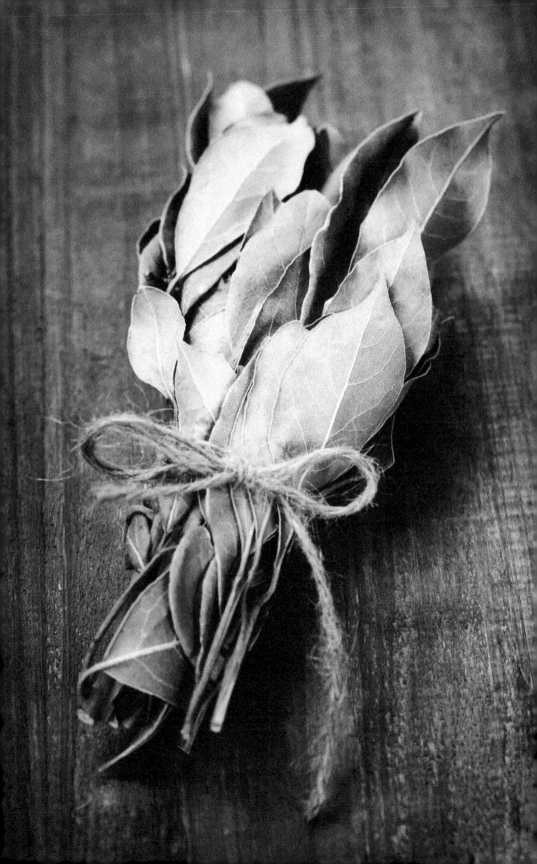

- In a bath
- In a cream blend
- In a massage oil blend
- In a vaporizer or diffuser

COMPLEMENTARY OILS

- Bergamot
- Cedarwood
- Cinnamon
- Clove
- Coriander
- Eucalyptus
- Frankincense
- Lavender
- Lemon
- Myrrh
- Neroli
- Orange
- Peppermint
- Petitgrain
- Rose
- Sandalwood
- Vetiver

WHAT TO WATCH OUT FOR

Do not use benzoin oil in large amounts—it can have a sedative effect.

May act as a sedative

Bergamot *Citrus aurantium*

Native to Southeast Asia, bergamot oil has a fresh citrusy scent and is one of the most popular essential oils. The source plant now grows in Europe, the Ivory Coast, Morocco, Tunisia, and Algeria. The oil can be obtained either through cold-pressing the rind or through steam distillation of the whole ripe fruit.

WHAT IT'S USED FOR

- Anorexia
- Anxiety
- Cystitis
- Depression
- Infections
- Psoriasis and eczema
- Stress
- Tension
- Urinary tract infections
- Wounds and cuts

- In a bath
- In a cream blend (for wounds, cuts, and skin conditions)
- In a massage oil blend
- In a vaporizer or diffuser

COMPLEMENTARY OILS

- Basil
- Benzoin
- Black pepper
- Cajeput
- Carrot seed
- Cedarwood
- Chamomile (German)
- Chamomile (Roman)
- Citronella
- Clary sage
- Coriander
- Cypress
- Dill
- Frankincense
- Geranium
- Ginger
- Grapefruit
- Helichrysum
- Jasmine
- Juniper berry
- Lavandin
- Lavender
- Marjoram
- Neroli
- Nutmeg
- Orange
- Palma rosa
- Patchouli
- Petitgrain
- Rose geranium
- Rosemary
- Rosewood
- Sage
- Sandalwood
- Tangerine/mandarin
- Thyme
- Vetiver
- Ylang-ylang

WHAT TO WATCH OUT FOR

Bergamot oil obtained through cold-pressing is a photosensitizing oil, so don't use it if you expect to be out in the sun within 12 hours of application, and never add bergamot oil to a tanning or sunscreen blend. Oils obtained by cold-pressing don't last long, so they need to be used within six months.

Avoid exposure to sunlight for 12 hours after use

May cause skin irritation

Use within six months of purchase date

Black Pepper *Piper nigrum*

Sharp and strong-smelling, with spicy overtones, black pepper oil comes mostly from Singapore, India, and Malaysia. The oil is produced through steam distillation of the plant's unripe fruit—the black peppercorns.

WHAT IT'S USED FOR

- Anorexia
- Arthritis
- Circulatory issues
- Colds and flu
- Constipation
- Exhaustion
- Fever
- Indigestion
- Muscle pain

HOW IT'S USED

- In a bath
- In a cream blend
- In a massage oil blend
- In a vaporizer or diffuser

COMPLEMENTARY OILS

- Basil
- Bergamot
- Cassia
- Clary sage
- Clove
- Coriander
- Fennel
- Frankincense
- Geranium
- Ginger
- Grapefruit
- Lavender
- Lemon
- Lime
- Nutmeg
- Orange
- Sage
- Sandalwood
- Tangerine/mandarin
- Ylang-ylang

Black pepper oil may irritate the skin. Too much black pepper oil can overwork the kidneys. Pregnant women should avoid black pepper oil.

Do not use during pregnancy

May cause skin irritation

Cajeput *Melaleuca cajuputi*

Also known as *cajuput, kayaputi, white wood, weeping tea tree*, and *weeping paperback*, cajeput has a sweet scent and is considered an effective repellent of lice and fleas. The tree grows on the Malayan coastal plains, and the oil is produced through steam distillation of the tree's leaves and twigs.

WHAT IT'S USED FOR

- Acne
- Arthritis
- Asthma
- Bronchitis
- Colds
- Colic
- Digestive issues
- Fever
- Infections
- Laryngitis
- Muscle pain
- Psoriasis
- Sinusitis
- Urinary tract infections
- Vomiting

HOW IT'S USED

- In a bath
- In a cream blend
- In a massage oil blend
- In a vaporizer or diffuser

COMPLEMENTARY OILS

- Angelica
- Bergamot
- Clove
- Geranium
- Lavender
- Thyme

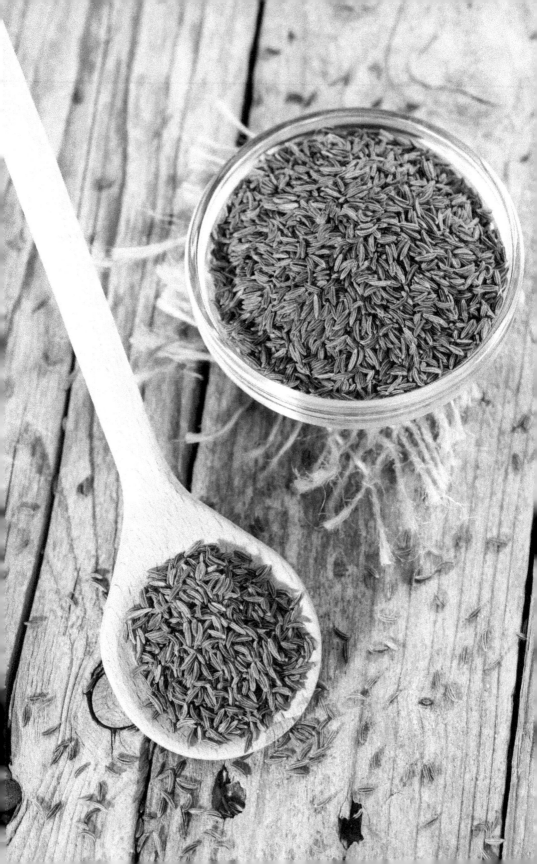

In high concentrations, cajeput oil may irritate the skin. It can also irritate mucous membranes.

Avoid contact with mucous membranes

May cause skin irritation

Caraway *Carum carvi, Apium carvi*

Sweet and peppery, caraway oil comes from a plant that originally grew only in Asia Minor but is now found in northern Europe, Russia, and Africa. It's also known as *meadow cumin*, and its use as a flavoring agent dates to ancient Egypt.

WHAT IT'S USED FOR

- Acne
- Asthma
- Bronchitis
- Bruises
- Colic
- Coughs
- Flatulence
- Itching
- Lactation issues
- Menstrual issues
- Mental fatigue
- Nervousness
- Scalp issues
- Stomach issues
- Urinary tract infections

HOW IT'S USED

- In a bath
- In a cream blend
- In a massage oil blend
- In a vaporizer or diffuser

COMPLEMENTARY OILS

- Aniseed
- Basil
- Cassia
- Coriander
- Dill
- Frankincense
- Ginger
- Lavender
- Orange

In high concentrations, caraway oil may irritate the skin.

May cause skin irritation

Carrot Seed *Daucus carota*

The well-known invasive plant Queen Anne's lace gives us carrot seed oil, with its earthy scent and many useful properties. The oil is produced from the plant's dried seeds through steam distillation.

WHAT IT'S USED FOR

- Arthritis
- Bronchitis
- Edema
- Flu
- Gout
- Liver issues

HOW IT'S USED

- In a bath
- In a cream blend or lotion blend
- In a massage oil blend
- In a vaporizer or diffuser

COMPLEMENTARY OILS

- Bergamot
- Bitter orange
- Cedarwood
- Geranium
- Grapefruit
- Lavender
- Lemon
- Lime
- Orange
- Rose geranium
- Tangerine/mandarin

WHAT TO WATCH OUT FOR

Although it is generally considered safe, pregnant women should avoid carrot seed oil.

Do not use during pregnancy

Cassia *Cinnamomum cassia*

Also known as *cassia bark* and *Chinese cinnamon*, cassia is often used as a powdered spice for curries in India, where it has earned the name *false cinnamon*. The essential oil is produced through steam distillation of the plant's leaves, bark, and twigs.

WHAT IT'S USED FOR

- Arthritis
- Colds and flu
- Colic
- Diarrhea
- Digestive issues
- Fever
- Flatulence
- Nausea

HOW IT'S USED

- In a vaporizer
- In a cream blend

COMPLEMENTARY OILS

- Balsam
- Black pepper
- Caraway
- Coriander
- Frankincense
- Geranium
- Ginger
- Nutmeg
- Rosemary

WHAT TO WATCH OUT FOR

Do not use cassia oil in a massage oil blend—it irritates the skin and mucous membranes. When using cassia oil in a cream, blend no more than 1 drop per ounce of cream to avoid irritating your skin. Pregnant women should avoid cassia oil.

Do not use during pregnancy

May cause skin irritation

Avoid contact with mucous membranes

Cedarwood *Juniperus virginiana*

The ancient Egyptians created the first essential oil from Lebanon cedar, a close relative of the cedarwood tree. Native Americans used cedarwood oil in medicinal applications as well as in purification rites. Today's cedarwood oil is steam-distilled from wood chips and sawdust.

WHAT IT'S USED FOR

- Anxiety
- Arthritis
- Bronchial congestion
- Itching
- Stress
- Tension
- Urinary tract infections

HOW IT'S USED

- In a bath
- In a cream blend
- In a massage oil blend
- In a vaporizer or diffuser

COMPLEMENTARY OILS

- Aniseed
- Basil
- Bay
- Benzoin
- Bergamot
- Carrot seed
- Cinnamon
- Cypress
- Frankincense
- Geranium
- Jasmine
- Juniper berry
- Lavender
- Lemon
- Lemongrass
- Marjoram
- Neroli
- Pine
- Rose
- Rose geranium
- Rosemary

WHAT TO WATCH OUT FOR

In high concentrations, cedarwood oil may be irritating to the skin. Pregnant women should avoid cedarwood oil.

Do not use during pregnancy

May cause skin irritation

Chamomile (German) *Matricaria chamomilla*

German chamomile, an earthy sweet-smelling herb, actually comes from France, Hungary, eastern Europe, and Egypt. It's also known as *blue chamomile, Hungarian chamomile*, and *single chamomile*. The oil produced from the plant is dark blue.

WHAT IT'S USED FOR

- Allergies
- Anxiety
- Eczema
- Gall bladder issues
- Inflammation
- Liver issues
- Menopausal symptoms
- Menstrual issues
- Pain
- Psoriasis
- Urinary stones

HOW IT'S USED

- In a bath
- In a cream blend or lotion blend
- In a massage oil blend
- In a vaporizer or diffuser

COMPLEMENTARY OILS

- Bergamot
- Clary sage
- Geranium
- Grapefruit
- Jasmine
- Lavender
- Lemon
- Rose
- Tea tree
- Ylang-ylang

WHAT TO WATCH OUT FOR

Because it can stimulate menstrual flow, pregnant women should avoid German chamomile oil.

Do not use during pregnancy

Chamomile (Roman)

Anthemis nobilis, Chamaemelum nobile

Roman chamomile, also known as *English chamomile,* differs in scent and appearance from German chamomile. Its fragrance evokes apples, and its color is light blue. The oil is produced through steam distillation of the herb's flowers.

WHAT IT'S USED FOR

- Abdominal pain
- Agitation in children
- Asthma
- Gall bladder issues
- Hay fever
- Itching
- Premenstrual symptoms
- Psoriasis
- Skin rashes
- Wounds

HOW IT'S USED

- In a bath
- In a cream blend or lotion blend
- In a massage oil blend
- In a vaporizer or diffuser

COMPLEMENTARY OILS

- Bergamot
- Clary sage
- Geranium
- Grapefruit
- Jasmine
- Lavender
- Lemon
- Melissa
- Rose
- Tea tree
- Ylang-ylang

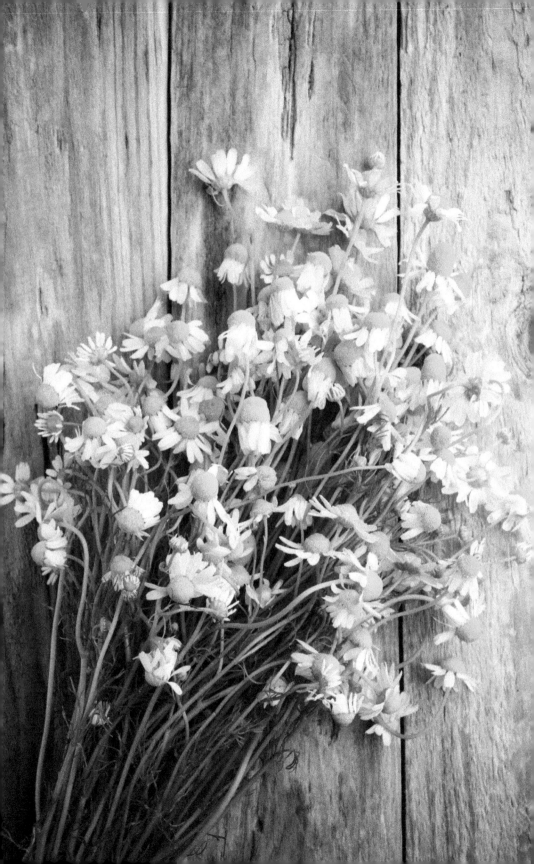

Because it can stimulate menstrual flow, pregnant women should avoid Roman chamomile oil.

Do not use during pregnancy

Cinnamon *Cinnamomum zeylanicum*

True cinnamon, also known as *Ceylon cinnamon, Madagascar cinnamon*, and *Seychelles cinnamon*, comes from Indonesia, Sri Lanka, and India. Most cinnamon oil used in the West is steam-distilled from the leaves of the cinnamon plant rather than from its bark, since the leaves have a more delicate scent and texture. The powdered cinnamon used in cooking comes from the plant's bark.

WHAT IT'S USED FOR

- Arthritis
- Colds and flu
- Digestive issues
- Menstrual issues
- Respiratory infections

HOW IT'S USED

- In a bath
- In a cream blend or lotion blend
- In a massage oil blend
- In a vaporizer or diffuser

COMPLEMENTARY OILS

- Benzoin
- Cardamom
- Cedarwood
- Clove
- Coriander
- Frankincense
- Ginger
- Grapefruit
- Lavender
- Orange
- Rosemary
- Tangerine/mandarin
- Tea tree
- Thyme

Cinnamon oil can irritate the skin. Because it can stimulate menstrual flow, pregnant women should avoid cinnamon oil.

Do not use during pregnancy

May cause skin irritation

Citronella *Cymbopogon nardus*

This grass is native to Sri Lanka and Java, but you're probably familiar with its sweet lemony smell if you've ever spent time on an outdoor patio where mosquitoes were fierce, since the steam-distilled essential oil is an effective insecticide. Citronella oil also serves as an antiseptic, a tonic, and an air freshener.

WHAT IT'S USED FOR

- Colds and flu

HOW IT'S USED

- In a cream blend or lotion blend
- In a vaporizer or diffuser

COMPLEMENTARY OILS

- Bergamot
- Geranium
- Lavandin
- Lavender
- Lemon
- Pine
- Rose geranium
- Rosemary

WHAT TO WATCH OUT FOR

Citronella oil may irritate the skin.

May cause skin irritation

Clary Sage *Salvia sclarea*

The source plant of versatile clary sage oil is known around the world by a number of names—*clary wort, muscatel sage, oculus Christi, clear eye, see bright,* and *eye bright* (the latter should not be confused with an unrelated plant called *eyebright,* of the genus *Euphrasia*). Clary sage comes from southern Europe, and the oil is produced through steam distillation of the plant's flowers and leaves.

WHAT IT'S USED FOR

- Depression
- Digestive disorders
- Insomnia
- Kidney issues
- Labor-related issues
- Menopausal symptoms
- Menstrual issues
- Muscle pain
- Stress
- Tension

HOW IT'S USED

- In a bath
- In a cream blend or lotion blend
- In a massage oil blend
- In a vaporizer or diffuser

COMPLEMENTARY OILS

- Bergamot
- Bitter orange
- Black pepper
- Chamomile (German)
- Chamomile (Roman)
- Clove
- Cypress
- Frankincense
- Geranium
- Grapefruit
- Helichrysum
- Hyssop
- Jasmine
- Juniper berry
- Lavandin
- Lavender
- Lemon
- Lime
- Nutmeg
- Orange
- Patchouli
- Pine
- Rose geranium
- Sandalwood
- Spikenard
- Tagetes
- Tangerine/mandarin
- Tea tree

Don't use clary sage oil in combination with alcoholic beverages—it can exaggerate the effects. Clary sage oil can cause a headache if too much is inhaled. Pregnant women should avoid clary sage oil.

Do not use during pregnancy

Do not use while consuming alcohol

May cause headache

Clove *Eugenia caryophyllata*

The warm, spicy aroma that comes from the buds of the clove tree is familiar to cooks and pastry chefs everywhere. Clove oil comes from Indonesia and the Melaka Islands, where the buds are beaten from the trees and dried for water distillation. It's also considered an effective moth repellent.

WHAT IT'S USED FOR

- Acne
- Arthritis
- Asthma
- Bruises
- Burns
- Cuts and scrapes
- Digestive upsets
- Pain

HOW IT'S USED

- In a cream blend or lotion blend
- In a massage oil blend
- In a vaporizer or diffuser

COMPLEMENTARY OILS

- Basil
- Benzoin
- Black pepper
- Cajeput
- Cinnamon
- Clary sage
- Ginger
- Lavender

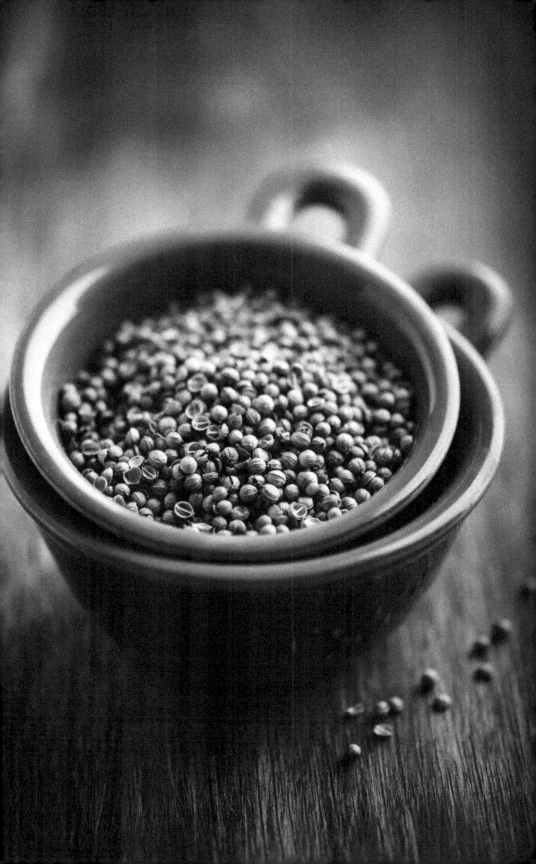

- Myrrh
- Orange
- Rose
- Sandalwood
- Tangerine/mandarin
- Tea tree

Clove oil can irritate the skin and mucous membranes, so use it only in low concentrations. Pregnant women should avoid clove oil.

Avoid contact with mucous membranes

Do not use during pregnancy

May cause skin irritation

Coriander *Coriandrum sativum*

Coriander oil, coriander seed oil, and Chinese parsley oil are all the same thing: a sweet, spicy oil that comes from an herb native to Morocco. It's the seeds that give coriander its sweet flavor and scent—a leaf crushed between the fingers yields a bitter smell. Some say the ancient Egyptians discovered coriander as an aphrodisiac. If so, it's not clear that the news ever reached medieval France, where nuns of the Carmelite order used the herb to flavor their water. These days, coriander flavors Benedictine and Chartreuse liqueurs.

WHAT IT'S USED FOR

- Arthritis
- Colds and flu
- Cramps
- Flatulence
- Mental fatigue
- Migraine and other types of headaches
- Muscle spasms
- Stress
- Tension

HOW IT'S USED

- In a bath
- In a cream blend or lotion blend
- In a massage oil blend
- In a vaporizer or diffuser

- Aniseed
- Bay
- Benzoin
- Bergamot
- Black pepper
- Caraway
- Cassia
- Cinnamon
- Ginger
- Grapefruit
- Lemon
- Lemongrass
- Neroli
- Niaouli
- Orange

WHAT TO WATCH OUT FOR

Large doses of coriander can have a sedative effect.

May act as a sedative

Cypress *Cupressus sempervirens*

The oil of this Mediterranean evergreen lends its woodsy scent to aftershave lotions and other cosmetics, and the wood has been used for centuries in building and ship construction. Cypress needles and twigs furnish the oil, which is produced through steam distillation.

WHAT IT'S USED FOR

- Agitation
- Asthma
- Bleeding
- Coughs and bronchitis
- Emphysema
- Excessive perspiration
- Flu
- Fluid retention
- Hemorrhoids
- Varicose veins
- Whooping cough

HOW IT'S USED

- In a bath
- In a cream blend or lotion blend

- In a cold pack
- In a foot bath
- In a massage oil blend
- In a vaporizer or diffuser

- Bergamot
- Bitter orange
- Clary sage
- Frankincense
- Grapefruit
- Juniper berry
- Lavender
- Lemon
- Lime
- Marjoram
- Nutmeg
- Orange
- Pine
- Rosemary
- Sandalwood
- Tangerine/mandarin

WHAT TO WATCH OUT FOR

Before using cypress oil for massage, perform a skin patch text. Pregnant women should avoid cypress oil.

Do not use during pregnancy

May cause skin irritation

Dill *Anethum sowa*

Dill, with its fresh aroma of newly mowed grass, comes from southwest Asia. This herb's uses in the kitchen have made it a staple ingredient for most cooks. The oil, extracted from the herb and its seeds through steam distillation, has a calming effect on mind and body.

WHAT IT'S USED FOR

- Digestive issues
- Headaches
- Lactation issues
- Stress
- Tension
- Wounds

- In a bath
- In a cream blend or lotion blend
- In a massage oil blend
- In a vaporizer or diffuser

COMPLEMENTARY OILS

- Aniseed
- Bergamot
- Bitter orange
- Caraway
- Grapefruit
- Lemon
- Lime
- Nutmeg
- Orange
- Tangerine/mandarin

WHAT TO WATCH OUT FOR

Dill oil is a photosensitizing oil, so don't use it if you expect to be out in the sun within 12 hours of application, and never add dill oil to a tanning or sunscreen blend. Pregnant women should avoid dill oil.

Avoid exposure to sunlight for 12 hours after use

Do not use during pregnancy

May cause skin irritation

Eucalyptus *Eucalyptus globulus, E. radiata*

Blue gum and *Tasmanian blue gum* are variant names for eucalyptus, the oil with the scent that hovers between mint, fresh leaves, and clean air. Its menthol-like properties make it one of the most popular exports from Australia, where the eucalyptus tree grows in abundance, and the oil's uses range from clearing the respiratory tract to healing ulcers.

WHAT IT'S USED FOR

- Chicken pox
- Circulatory issues
- Fever
- Inflammation

- Malaria
- Measles
- Migraine and other types of headaches
- Muscle aches and pains
- Respiratory ailments and infections
- Rheumatoid arthritis

HOW IT'S USED

- As a gargle
- In a bath
- In a cream blend or lotion blend
- In a massage oil blend
- In a vaporizer or diffuser
- In neat (undiluted) applications

COMPLEMENTARY OILS

- Bay
- Benzoin
- Lavender
- Lemon
- Lemongrass
- Marjoram
- Peppermint
- Pine
- Spearmint
- Thyme

WHAT TO WATCH OUT FOR

People with high blood pressure and epilepsy should avoid eucalyptus oil. Excessive use may cause headaches.

Do not use if you have epilepsy

Do not use if you have high blood pressure

May cause headaches

Fennel *Foeniculum vulgare*

The spicy, herblike scent of fennel attracted interest in the ancient civilizations of Egypt, Rome, and China, where the plant's use was believed to bestow a long life and ward off evil spirits. The oil is produced from the seeds through steam distillation.

WHAT IT'S USED FOR

- Anorexia
- Cellulite
- Digestive issues
- Dysplasia
- Hiccups
- Liver issues
- Obesity
- Skin issues
- Spleen issues

HOW IT'S USED

- In a bath
- In a cream blend or lotion blend
- In a massage oil blend
- In a vaporizer or diffuser

COMPLEMENTARY OILS

- Aniseed
- Basil
- Black pepper
- Geranium
- Lavender
- Lemon
- Myrrh
- Niaouli
- Rose
- Sandalwood

WHAT TO WATCH OUT FOR

In large doses, fennel can have a narcotic effect. Pregnant women, people with estrogen-linked cancers, breast-feeding mothers, and women with endometriosis should avoid fennel.

Do not use during pregnancy or while nursing

Do not use if you have an estrogen-linked cancer

Do not use if you have endometriosis

May act as a sedative

Frankincense *Boswellia carteri*

Known as *olibanum* and *gum thus* as well as by the name made famous in the New Testament story of the three wise men, frankincense mixes notes of wood resin and musk with a menthol-like freshness. Not surprisingly, frankincense comes from the Middle East. A complex process of extracting the plant's gum leads to the steam distillation of frankincense oil.

WHAT IT'S USED FOR

- Agitation during labor and delivery
- Anxiety
- Arthritis
- Asthma
- Excessive volume or rapidity of menstrual flow
- Skin inflammation and wounds
- Stress
- Urinary tract issues
- Wounds

HOW IT'S USED

- As a wash
- In a bath
- In a cream blend or lotion blend
- In a massage oil blend
- In a vaporizer or diffuser
- In a warm compress

COMPLEMENTARY OILS

- Benzoin
- Bergamot
- Black pepper
- Caraway
- Cassia
- Cedarwood
- Cinnamon
- Clary sage
- Cypress
- Ginger
- Grapefruit
- Lavender
- Lemon
- Melissa
- Orange
- Pine
- Sandalwood
- Tangerine/mandarin

Frankincense is not associated with any specific warnings.

Geranium *Pelargonium odorantissimum*

This oil has a floral scent, with just a hint of apples and mint. The original geraniums came from South Africa, the island of Réunion, Madagascar, Egypt, and Morocco. There are hundreds of varieties of geraniums throughout the world, but geranium oil comes from only 10 of them. The oil is produced from the plant's leaves and stalks through steam distillation.

WHAT IT'S USED FOR

- Breast engorgement
- Circulatory issues
- Head lice
- Neuralgia
- Premenstrual issues
- Ringworm
- Skin issues
- Sore throat and tonsillitis
- Stress
- Ulcers

HOW IT'S USED

- As a shampoo
- In a bath
- In a cream blend or lotion blend
- In a massage oil blend
- In a vaporizer or diffuser

COMPLEMENTARY OILS

- Allspice
- Angelica
- Basil
- Bay
- Bergamot
- Black pepper
- Cajeput
- Carrot seed
- Cassia
- Cedarwood
- Chamomile (German)
- Chamomile (Roman)
- Citronella
- Clary sage
- Fennel
- Grapefruit

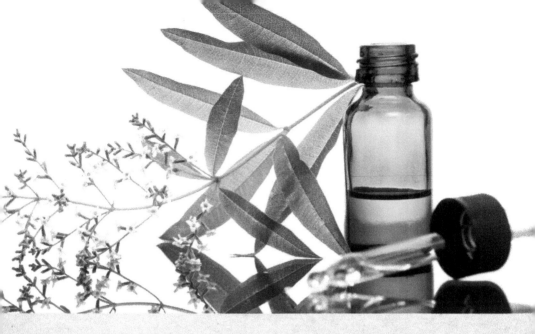

HANDLE WITH CARE
Essential Oil Safety

Some essential oils are believed to pose no particular dangers, but all essential oils should be handled carefully. Always take the following precautions, even with oils considered to be generally safe:

1. If you accidentally get some essential oil into your eyes, *do not flush your eyes with water*. Instead, flush them with vegetable oil or cold milk to dilute the essential oil (if you wear contact lenses, be sure to remove them first). Seek medical attention right away if stinging lasts for more than a few minutes.
2. If you accidentally swallow some essential oil, *do not induce vomiting*. Rinse your mouth with cold milk or water to dilute the essential oil, and seek immediate medical attention.
3. If your skin becomes irritated by an essential oil, remove any contaminated clothing, and wash the irritated area with plenty of soap and water. Seek medical attention if skin irritation continues.
4. Avoid overexposure—*do not inhale essential oils casually*. After inhaling an essential oil, move immediately to a source of fresh air if you experience trouble breathing, dizziness, or nausea.

- Hyssop
- Jasmine
- Juniper berry
- Lavender
- Lemon
- Lemongrass
- Lime
- Melissa
- Neroli
- Nutmeg
- Orange
- Palma rosa
- Patchouli
- Petitgrain
- Rose
- Rosemary
- Sandalwood
- Tea tree

WHAT TO WATCH OUT FOR

Because it affects the endocrine system, pregnant women should avoid geranium oil.

Do not use during pregnancy

Ginger *Zingiberaceae officinale*

Ginger is claimed as a native plant in regions as diverse as India, China, Africa, and the West Indies. Sanskrit and Chinese texts make reference to ginger oil, and the ancient Greeks, Romans, and Arabians are said to have used it for a wide range of ailments. Ginger oil, reputed to possess both aphrodisiac and curative properties, is produced through steam distillation of the plant's root, which is dried with the skin on and ground before the distillation process begins.

WHAT IT'S USED FOR

- Catarrh
- Chills and fever
- Colds
- Digestive issues
- Motion sickness
- Nausea
- Sinusitis
- Skin sores
- Sore throat

- As a neat (undiluted) application on a handkerchief
- In a bath
- In a cream blend or lotion blend
- In a vaporizer or diffuser
- In a warm compress

- Allspice
- Basil
- Bay
- Bergamot
- Bitter orange
- Black pepper
- Caraway
- Cassia
- Cinnamon
- Clove
- Coriander
- Frankincense
- Grapefruit
- Lemon
- Lime
- Neroli
- Orange
- Rose
- Sandalwood
- Tangerine/mandarin
- Ylang-ylang

Ginger oil can irritate the skin. Ginger oil is a photosensitizing oil, so don't use it if you expect to be out in the sun within 12 hours of application, and never add ginger oil to a tanning or sunscreen blend.

Avoid exposure to sunlight for 12 hours after use

May cause skin irritation

Grapefruit *Citrus paradisi, C. racemosa*

Bright and refreshing grapefruit oil originally came from the fruit of a tree native to Asia, but grapefruit trees are now cultivated throughout the western hemisphere. The oil can be obtained either through cold-pressing of the rind or through steam distillation of the whole ripe fruit, but these days grapefruit oil is virtually always obtained through cold-pressing.

- Acne
- Cellulite
- Colds and flu
- Depression
- Hair loss
- Immunosuppression
- Muscle fatigue
- Obesity
- Stress
- Urine retention

HOW IT'S USED

- As a wash
- In a bath
- In a cream blend or lotion blend
- In a massage oil blend
- In a vaporizer or diffuser

COMPLEMENTARY OILS

- Basil
- Bergamot
- Black pepper
- Carrot seed
- Chamomile (German)
- Chamomile (Roman)
- Cinnamon
- Clary sage
- Coriander
- Cypress
- Dill
- Frankincense
- Geranium
- Ginger
- Jasmine
- Juniper berry
- Lavender
- Neroli
- Palma rosa
- Rose geranium
- Rosewood
- Thyme
- Vetiver
- Ylang-ylang

WHAT TO WATCH OUT FOR

Grapefruit oil obtained through cold-pressing is a photosensitizing oil, so don't use it if you expect to be out in the sun within 12 hours of application, and never add grapefruit oil to a tanning or sunscreen blend. Oils obtained by cold-pressing don't last long, so they need to be used within six months.

Avoid exposure to sunlight for 12 hours after use

May cause skin irritation

Use within six months of purchase date

Helichrysum *Helichrysum angustifolium*

Everlasting oil, immortelle, and *St. John's herb* are alternate names for this versatile evergreen herb with its robust fragrance. The oil is produced through steam distillation of the plant's dark-yellow flowers, which must be quickly harvested and processed immediately. Helichrysum and its oil have been used in Europe since the Middle Ages.

WHAT IT'S USED FOR

- Arthritis
- Circulatory issues
- Digestive issues
- Respiratory issues
- Scars and other skin lesions

HOW IT'S USED

- In a bath
- In a cream blend or lotion blend
- In a massage oil blend
- In a vaporizer

COMPLEMENTARY OILS

- Bergamot
- Clary sage
- Lavender
- Rosewood
- Tangerine/mandarin

WHAT TO WATCH OUT FOR

Do not use this oil with children younger than 12.

Not safe for children under 12

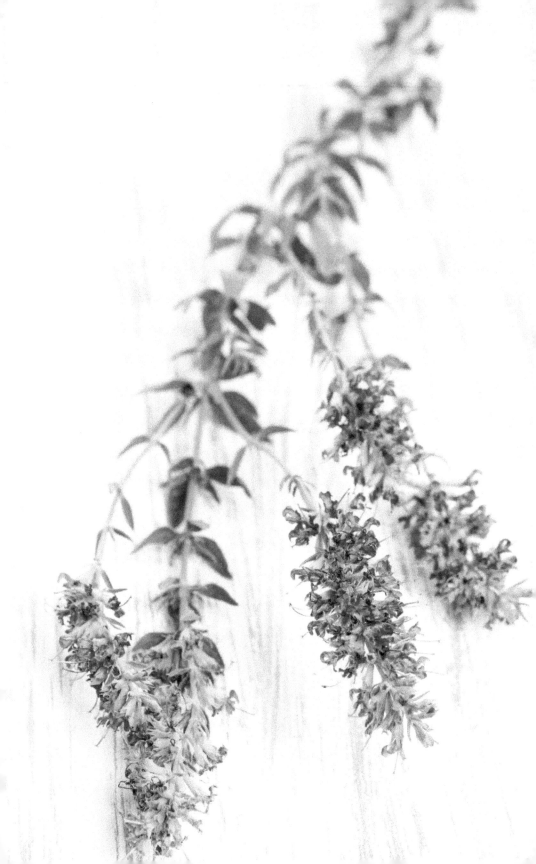

Hyssop   *Hyssopus officinalis*

Once known as *azob*, this pricey oil comes from a Mediterranean plant used in ancient Greece by Hippocrates. The Old Testament also contains references to *ezob* ("holy herb"), which was used for purification. By the 10th century CE, the Benedictine monks were using hyssop in their liqueurs.

WHAT IT'S USED FOR

- Anxiety
- Colds and flu
- Colic
- Fatigue
- Flatulence
- Fluid retention
- Genitourinary issues
- Indigestion
- Menstrual issues
- Respiratory issues

HOW IT'S USED

- In a bath
- In a cream blend or lotion blend
- In a massage oil blend
- In a vaporizer or diffuser

COMPLEMENTARY OILS

- Angelica
- Clary sage
- Geranium
- Melissa
- Orange
- Rosemary
- Tangerine/mandarin

WHAT TO WATCH OUT FOR

Hyssop oil contains pinocamphone, the neurotoxin found in early recipes for absinthe, so its use should be moderated. Pregnant women and people with epilepsy should avoid hyssop oil.

Do not use during pregnancy

Do not use if you have epilepsy

Jasmine *Jasminum grandiflorum*

Jasmine comes from plants that grow in France, Italy, Morocco, Egypt, China, Japan, and Turkey. Jasmine oil is produced through steam distillation of an absolute extracted from a concrete (see page 12 for more about absolute and concrete in solvent extraction).

WHAT IT'S USED FOR

- Depression
- Erectile dysfunction
- Labor-related issues
- Respiratory illnesses
- Scars
- Skin issues
- Stretch marks

HOW IT'S USED

- In a bath
- In a cream blend or lotion blend
- In a massage oil blend
- In a vaporizer or diffuser

COMPLEMENTARY OILS

- Bergamot
- Bitter orange
- Cedarwood
- Chamomile (German)
- Chamomile (Roman)
- Clary sage
- Geranium
- Grapefruit
- Lavandin
- Lemon
- Lemongrass
- Lime
- Neroli
- Orange
- Rose
- Rose geranium
- Sandalwood
- Spearmint
- Tagetes
- Tangerine/mandarin
- Vetiver

WHAT TO WATCH OUT FOR

Jasmine oil can cause an allergic reaction. Because it stimulates menstrual flow, pregnant women should avoid jasmine oil. This oil can have a sedative effect.

268   Essential Oils and Aromatherapy: An Introductory Guide

Do not use during pregnancy

May act as a sedative

May cause an allergic reaction

Juniper Berry *Juniperus communis*

Varieties of juniper live all over the world, and the plant's essential oil may come from one of several continents, including North America. The oil is also used to flavor gin.

WHAT IT'S USED FOR

- Arthritis
- Cellulite
- Digestive issues
- Fluid retention
- Gout
- Menstrual issues
- Skin issues
- Stress
- Tension
- Urinary, prostate, and kidney issues

HOW IT'S USED

- In a bath
- In a cream blend or lotion blend
- In a massage oil blend
- In a vaporizer or diffuser
- In a warm compress

COMPLEMENTARY OILS

- Bergamot
- Cedarwood
- Clary sage
- Cypress
- Geranium
- Grapefruit
- Lavandin
- Lavender
- Lemongrass
- Lime
- Vetiver

Because it stimulates the muscles of the uterus, pregnant women should avoid juniper oil. Juniper berry is a natural diuretic, so it is good for people with healthy kidneys who want to increase urination or combat water retention. However, it can over-stimulate the kidneys, and should not be used when kidneys are inflamed or infected, or by people with kidney disease.

Do not use during pregnancy

Do not use if you have kidney disease

Lavandin *Lavandula hybrida, L. hortensis*

Often confused with lavender, this plant is larger and is often called *bastard lavender* because it comes from a hybrid of true lavender and spike lavender. Lavandin grows in France and is used extensively in manufacturing perfumes and other scented products.

WHAT IT'S USED FOR

- Colds and flu
- Coughs
- Muscle pain and stiffness

HOW IT'S USED

- In a vaporizer or diffuser
- In a bath
- In a cream blend or lotion blend

COMPLEMENTARY OILS

- Bergamot
- Cinnamon
- Citronella
- Clary sage
- Jasmine
- Juniper berry
- Patchouli
- Pine
- Rosemary
- Thyme

Lavandin is not associated with any specific warnings.

Lavender *Lavandula angustifolia, L. officinalis, L. spica*

The single most universal and versatile essential oil, lavender gained its reputation for calming and curative powers in the days of the Roman Empire, when it was used for bathing, strewn on floors as a room deodorizer, and stuffed into sachets to add fragrance to clothing and linens. The Romans transported lavender to England, and the woody plant became a worldwide favorite.

WHAT IT'S USED FOR

- Agitation
- Anxiety
- Minor burns
- Nausea and vomiting
- Pain
- Respiratory issues
- Skin blemishes and other skin issues

HOW IT'S USED

- As a neat (undiluted) application on a cotton ball
- In a bath
- In a cold pack
- In a cream blend or lotion blend
- In a massage oil blend
- In a vaporizer or diffuser

COMPLEMENTARY OILS

- Allspice
- Basil
- Bay
- Benzoin
- Bergamot
- Bitter orange
- Black pepper
- Cajeput
- Caraway
- Carrot seed
- Cedarwood
- Chamomile (German)
- Chamomile (Roman)
- Cinnamon
- Citronella
- Clary sage
- Clove
- Cypress

- Eucalyptus
- Fennel
- Frankincense
- Geranium
- Grapefruit
- Helichrysum
- Juniper berry
- Lemon
- Lemongrass
- Lemon verbena
- Lime
- Melissa
- Myrrh
- Neroli
- Niaouli
- Nutmeg
- Orange
- Patchouli
- Peppermint
- Petitgrain
- Pine
- Rose geranium
- Rosemary
- Sage
- Sandalwood
- Spearmint
- Spikenard
- Tagetes
- Tangerine/mandarin
- Tea tree
- Thyme
- Vetiver
- Ylang-ylang

WHAT TO WATCH OUT FOR

Stop using lavender oil if you experience an allergic reaction.

May cause an allergic reaction

Lemon *Citrus limonum*

Who doesn't know the sharp and sour yet pleasing scent of lemon? This fruit originated in India and found its way, over the centuries, to the warmest regions of Europe and the United States. The oil can be obtained either through cold-pressing of the rind or through steam distillation of the whole ripe fruit.

WHAT IT'S USED FOR

- Arthritis
- Cellulite
- Circulatory issues
- Constipation
- Fever
- Herpes
- High blood pressure
- Insect bites

- Migraine and other types of headaches
- Skin issues
- Throat infections

HOW IT'S USED

HOW IT'S USED

- In a cream blend or lotion blend
- In a massage oil blend
- In a vaporizer or diffuser

COMPLEMENTARY OILS

- Basil
- Bay
- Benzoin
- Black pepper
- Carrot seed
- Cedarwood
- Chamomile (German)
- Chamomile (Roman)
- Citronella
- Clary sage
- Coriander
- Cypress
- Dill
- Eucalyptus
- Fennel
- Frankincense
- Geranium
- Ginger
- Jasmine
- Lavender
- Neroli
- Peppermint
- Rose
- Rosewood
- Sage
- Sandalwood
- Spikenard
- Tagetes
- Tea tree
- Thyme

WHAT TO WATCH OUT FOR

Lemon oil obtained through cold-pressing is a photosensitizing oil, so don't use it if you expect to be out in the sun within 12 hours of application, and never add lemon oil to a tanning or sunscreen blend. Oils obtained by cold-pressing don't last long, so they need to be used within six months.

Avoid exposure to sunlight for 12 hours after use

May cause skin irritation

Use within six months of purchase date

Lemongrass *Cymbopogon citratus*

The fresh, clean scent of lemongrass oil comes from a plant that grows wild in India. Lemongrass adds a distinctive flavor to Indian and other southeast Asian cuisines, and the plant's essential oil is used as an insect repellent. Known as *choomana poolu* in India, lemongrass oil also goes by the names *Indian verbena oil* and *Indian melissa oil.*

WHAT IT'S USED FOR

- Acne
- Digestive issues
- Exhaustion
- Fever
- Headaches
- Infectious diseases
- Jet lag
- Muscle pain
- Respiratory infections
- Stress

HOW IT'S USED

- In a bath
- In a cream blend or lotion blend
- In a massage oil blend
- In a vaporizer or diffuser

COMPLEMENTARY OILS

- Basil
- Cedarwood
- Coriander
- Eucalyptus
- Geranium
- Jasmine
- Juniper berry
- Lavender
- Rosemary
- Tea tree

WHAT TO WATCH OUT FOR

Lemongrass oil may irritate the skin. Pregnant women should avoid lemongrass oil.

Do not use during pregnancy

May cause skin irritation

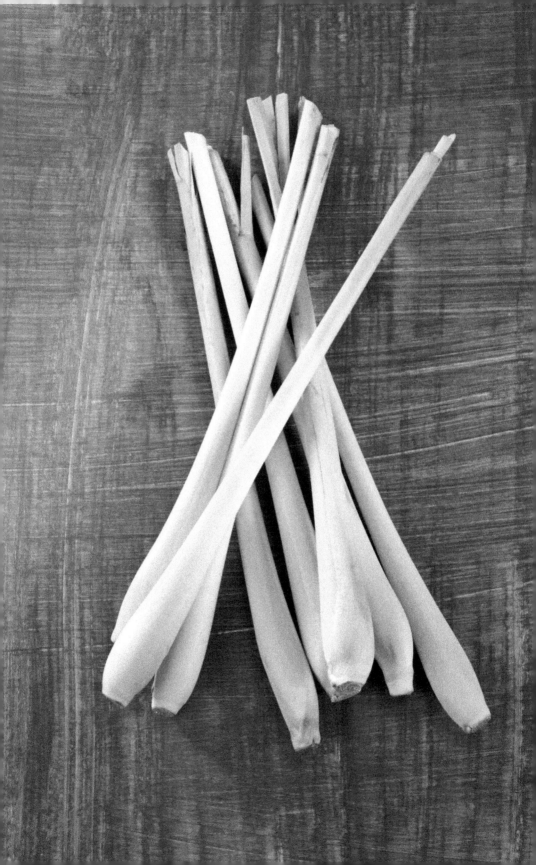

Lemon Verbena *Lippia citrodora, Aloysia triphylla*

A native of Chile, this mild, lemony oil comes from the leaves of a tall shrub. The leaves are harvested and used while they are fresh, and the oil is extracted through steam distillation.

WHAT IT'S USED FOR

- Depression
- Digestive issues
- Hangover
- Heart palpitations
- Liver issues
- Sexual dysfunction
- Stress

HOW IT'S USED

- In a bath
- In a cream blend or lotion blend
- In a massage oil blend
- In a vaporizer or diffuser

COMPLEMENTARY OILS

- Lemon
- Neroli
- Palma rosa

WHAT TO WATCH OUT FOR

Lemon verbena is a photosensitizing oil, so don't use it if you expect to be out in the sun within 12 hours of application, and never add lemon verbena oil to a tanning or sunscreen blend.

Avoid exposure to sunlight for 12 hours after use

May cause skin irritation

Lime *Citrus aurantiifolia*

The lime tree, native to Asia, is now also common in the warmer parts of Italy, the West Indies, and North and South America. The oil is considered to be an immunity booster and can be obtained either through cold-pressing of the fruit's rind or through steam distillation of the whole ripe fruit.

WHAT IT'S USED FOR

- Acne
- Arthritis
- Cellulite
- Circulatory issues
- Cuts and scrapes
- Fever
- Herpes
- Insect bites

HOW IT'S USED

- In a bath
- In a cream blend or lotion blend
- In a massage oil blend
- In a vaporizer or diffuser

COMPLEMENTARY OILS

- Black pepper
- Carrot seed
- Clary sage
- Cypress
- Dill
- Geranium
- Ginger
- Jasmine
- Juniper berry
- Lavender
- Neroli
- Niaouli
- Palma rosa
- Rose geranium
- Rosewood
- Ylang-ylang

WHAT TO WATCH OUT FOR

Lime oil obtained through cold-pressing is a photosensitizing oil, so don't use it if you expect to be out in the sun within 12 hours of application, and never add lime oil to a tanning or sunscreen blend. Oils obtained by cold-pressing don't last long, so they need to be used within six months.

Avoid exposure to sunlight for 12 hours after use

May cause skin irritation

Use within six months of purchase date

Mandarin

Citrus reticulate, C. nobilis, C. madurensis, C. unshiu, C. deliciosa

See *Tangerine*.

Marjoram *Origanum majorana*

Warm and spicy, marjoram essential oil comes from a Mediterranean herb used extensively in ancient Greece for its therapeutic and fragrant properties. The oil is produced from the plant's fresh and dried leaves through steam distillation.

WHAT IT'S USED FOR

- Anxiety
- Arthritis
- Diminished libido
- Hyperactivity
- Insomnia
- Menstrual issues
- Migraine and other types of headaches
- Muscle pain
- Respiratory issues
- Stress

HOW IT'S USED

- In a bath
- In a cream blend or lotion blend
- In a massage oil blend
- In a vaporizer or diffuser

COMPLEMENTARY OILS

- Basil
- Bergamot
- Cedarwood
- Cypress
- Eucalyptus
- Peppermint
- Tea tree

Because it can stimulate menstrual flow, pregnant women should avoid marjoram oil.

Do not use during pregnancy

Melissa *Melissa officinalis*

Melissa is also known as *lemon balm* and *bee balm*. As it happens, *melissa* is Greek for *honeybee*, the name of a tiny creature that loves this Mediterranean plant and its small pinkish flowers. Melissa essential oil is produced from the plant's flowers, leaves, and stems through steam distillation.

WHAT IT'S USED FOR

- Anxiety
- Cold sores
- Depression
- Digestive upsets
- Fever
- High blood pressure
- Migraine and other types of headaches

HOW IT'S USED

- In a bath
- In a cream blend or lotion blend
- In a massage oil blend
- In a vaporizer or diffuser

COMPLEMENTARY OILS

- Basil
- Chamomile (Roman)
- Frankincense
- Geranium
- Hyssop
- Lavender
- Rose
- Ylang-ylang

Use melissa oil only in low concentrations, since it can irritate the skin. Pregnant women should avoid melissa oil.

Do not use during pregnancy

May cause skin irritation

Myrrh *Commiphora myrrha, C. molmol, Balsamodendrum myrrha*

Myrrh essential oil comes from the gum resin of a tree that grows in Somalia and the Arab countries. Along with frankincense, myrrh is famous as one of the three gifts presented to the infant Jesus in Bethlehem by the three wise men of the New Testament. This versatile oil is produced from the plant's gum through steam distillation.

WHAT IT'S USED FOR

- Digestive issues
- Hemorrhoids
- Labor-related issues
- Menstrual issues
- Pulmonary congestion
- Sinusitis
- Skin issues

HOW IT'S USED

- In a bath
- In a cream blend or lotion blend
- In a cold pack
- In a massage oil blend
- In a vaporizer or diffuser

COMPLEMENTARY OILS

- Benzoin
- Clove
- Frankincense
- Lavender
- Patchouli
- Sandalwood
- Tagetes
- Tea tree

Myrrh oil can be toxic in large doses. Because it stimulates the muscles of the uterus, pregnant women should avoid myrrh oil.

Do not use during pregnancy

May be toxic if taken internally

Neroli   *Citrus aurantium*

This oil takes its name from a 17th-century Italian princess of Nerola, Anna Maria de la Trémoille, who used it as her trademark fragrance, although the oil may be better known as *orange blossom oil*. Whatever you want to call it, this is an unusually expensive oil, mainly because it takes half a ton of orange blossoms to produce a single pound of oil.

WHAT IT'S USED FOR

- Anxiety
- Depression
- Digestive issues
- Headaches
- Heart palpitations
- Insomnia
- Scars
- Stress
- Stretch marks
- Vertigo

HOW IT'S USED

- In a bath
- In a cream blend or lotion blend
- In a massage oil blend
- In a vaporizer or diffuser

COMPLEMENTARY OILS

- Basil
- Benzoin
- Bergamot
- Bitter orange
- Cedarwood
- Coriander
- Geranium
- Ginger
- Grapefruit
- Jasmine

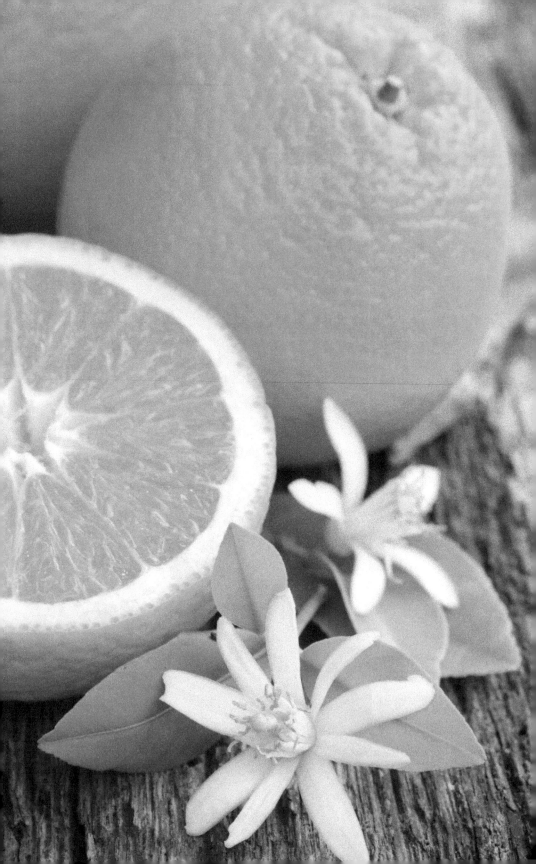

- Lavender
- Lemon
- Lemon verbena
- Lime
- Orange
- Rose geranium
- Rosemary
- Sandalwood
- Spikenard
- Tangerine/mandarin
- Ylang-ylang

WHAT TO WATCH OUT FOR

Neroli oil can be very relaxing, so it should not be used during operation of machinery or when clarity of thought is required.

May act as a sedative

Niaouli *Melaleuca viridiflora, M. quinquenervia*

This oil comes from the broad-leaved paperbark, an evergreen native to Australia. The oil's antibacterial properties came to light when it was discovered that the paperbark's leaves disinfect the ground where they fall. You may see niaouli essential oil listed as an ingredient in toothpaste and mouthwash. It's produced from the tree's leaves and twigs through steam distillation.

WHAT IT'S USED FOR

- Colds and flu
- Digestive tract infections
- Neuralgia
- Respiratory infections
- Urinary tract infections

HOW IT'S USED

- In a bath
- In a cream blend or lotion blend
- In a massage oil blend
- In a vaporizer or diffuser

- Coriander
- Fennel
- Lavender
- Lime
- Peppermint
- Pine

WHAT TO WATCH OUT FOR

Niaouli is not associated with any specific warnings.

Nutmeg *Myristica fragrans, M. officinalis, M. oromata, Nux moschata*

Nutmeg trees grow in the Molucca Islands, Penang, Java, and Sri Lanka. The tree's essential oil is produced from the kernel of its peachlike fruit through steam distillation.

WHAT IT'S USED FOR

- Anorexia
- Circulatory issues
- Constipation
- Digestive issues
- Fainting
- Gallstones
- Muscle pain
- Reproductive issues

HOW IT'S USED

- In a bath
- In a cream blend or lotion blend
- In a massage oil blend
- In a vaporizer or diffuser

COMPLEMENTARY OILS

- Black pepper
- Bergamot
- Cassia
- Clary sage
- Cypress
- Geranium
- Lavender
- Orange
- Rosemary
- Tangerine/mandarin
- Tea tree

Nutmeg oil may cause nausea, can be toxic in large doses, and can have a sedative effect. Pregnant women should avoid nutmeg oil.

Do not use during pregnancy

May act as a sedative

May be toxic if taken internally

Orange *Citrus sinensis, C. aurantium*

Often called *sweet orange oil,* this popular flavoring oil comes from trees native to China and now found in abundance in warmer climates of the United States. The oil can be obtained either through cold-pressing of the fruit's rind or through steam distillation of the whole ripe fruit.

WHAT IT'S USED FOR

- Digestive issues
- Fluid retention
- Immunosuppression
- Insomnia
- Stress
- Tension

HOW IT'S USED

- In a bath
- In a cream blend or lotion blend
- In a massage oil blend
- In a vaporizer

COMPLEMENTARY OILS

- Allspice
- Bay
- Benzoin
- Bergamot
- Black pepper
- Caraway
- Carrot seed
- Cinnamon
- Clary sage
- Clove
- Coriander
- Cypress

- Dill
- Frankincense
- Geranium
- Ginger
- Hyssop
- Jasmine
- Lavender
- Neroli
- Nutmeg
- Rose geranium
- Rosewood
- Sandalwood
- Vetiver

WHAT TO WATCH OUT FOR

Orange oil obtained through cold-pressing is a photosensitizing oil, so don't use it if you expect to be out in the sun within 12 hours of application, and never add orange oil to a tanning or sunscreen blend. Oils obtained by cold-pressing don't last long, so they need to be used within six months.

Avoid exposure to sunlight for 12 hours after use

May cause skin irritation

Use within six months of purchase date

Palma Rosa *Cymbopogon martinii*

You may find this oil labeled *East Indian geranium* or *Turkish geranium*, and it may be called *rosha* or *motia* in India. Palma rosa oil is extracted from one of two varieties (*motia* or *sofia*) of a grass that grows wild in southeast Asia, and the oil you purchase may be from either plant.

WHAT IT'S USED FOR

- Acne
- Aging skin
- Anorexia
- Athlete's foot
- Digestive issues
- Exhaustion
- Fever
- Muscle stiffness
- Stress

- As a wash
- In a bath
- In a cream blend or lotion blend
- In a massage oil blend
- In neat (undiluted) applications
- In a vaporizer or diffuser

COMPLEMENTARY OILS

- Bergamot
- Geranium
- Grapefruit
- Lemon verbena
- Lime
- Petitgrain
- Rose
- Rosemary
- Ylang-ylang

WHAT TO WATCH OUT FOR

Palma rosa oil may irritate the skin. Pregnant women should avoid palma rosa oil.

Do not use during pregnancy

May cause skin irritation

Patchouli *Pogostemon cablin, P. patchouli*

Musky, sweet-smelling patchouli oil comes from a plant native to India and Malaysia and has been used for centuries to repel moths and bedbugs. The oil is produced from the plant's young dried leaves through steam distillation.

WHAT IT'S USED FOR

- Acne
- Aging skin
- Anxiety
- Depression
- Diminished libido
- Fluid retention
- Infections
- Insect bite
- Wounds

- In a bath
- In a cream blend or lotion blend
- In a massage oil blend
- In a vaporizer or diffuser
- In neat (undiluted) applications

COMPLEMENTARY OILS

- Allspice
- Bergamot
- Clary sage
- Geranium
- Lavandin
- Lavender
- Myrrh
- Spikenard

WHAT TO WATCH OUT FOR

Inhaling too much patchouli oil may cause loss of appetite.

Peppermint *Mentha piperita*

Peppermint, originally from the Mediterranean region, is now culti-vated in the United States, Japan, Great Britain, and Italy. It spreads by way of underground runners, so it's an easy plant to grow. The oil is produced from the whole plant through steam distillation.

WHAT IT'S USED FOR

- Depression
- Digestive issues
- Menstrual issues
- Mental fatigue
- Migraine and other types of headaches
- Muscle pains
- Nausea
- Neuralgia
- Respiratory illnesses
- Skin irritation and inflammation
- Stress
- Sunburn
- Vertigo

- In a bath
- In a cream blend or lotion blend
- In a massage oil blend
- In a vaporizer or diffuser

COMPLEMENTARY OILS

- Benzoin
- Eucalyptus
- Lavender
- Lemon
- Marjoram
- Niaouli
- Rosemary

WHAT TO WATCH OUT FOR

Peppermint oil may irritate the skin. Peppermint oil can also irritate mucous membranes. Do not use peppermint oil around your eyes. Pregnant women should avoid peppermint oil, and it should not be used with children younger than seven.

Avoid contact with eyes

Avoid contact with mucous membranes

Do not use during pregnancy

May cause skin irritation

Not safe for children under 7

Petitgrain *Citrus aurantium, C. bigardia, Petitgrain bigarade*

Petitgrain oil, an oil obtained from the orange tree, comes from the tree's leaves and twigs rather than from its fruit (the source of orange oil) or its blossoms (the source of neroli oil). The complex aroma of petitgrain oil unites woody and floral notes.

- Acne
- Anger
- Exhaustion
- Insomnia
- Oily skin
- Stress

HOW IT'S USED

- In a bath
- In a cream blend or lotion blend
- In a massage oil blend
- In a vaporizer or diffuser

COMPLEMENTARY OILS

- Aniseed
- Benzoin
- Bergamot
- Lavender
- Geranium
- Palma rosa
- Rosewood
- Sandalwood

WHAT TO WATCH OUT FOR

Petitgrain is not associated with any specific warnings.

Pine *Pinus sylvestris*

Pine essential oil is produced on several continents. The pine oil distilled in the United States is generally collected from the Scotch pine, but some US distillers use other varieties. This crisp, fresh oil is produced from the tree's twigs and buds through steam distillation.

WHAT IT'S USED FOR

- Arthritis
- Cuts and scrapes
- Excessive perspiration
- Fatigue
- Gout
- Insect bites
- Muscle aches
- Respiratory issues
- Urinary tract issues

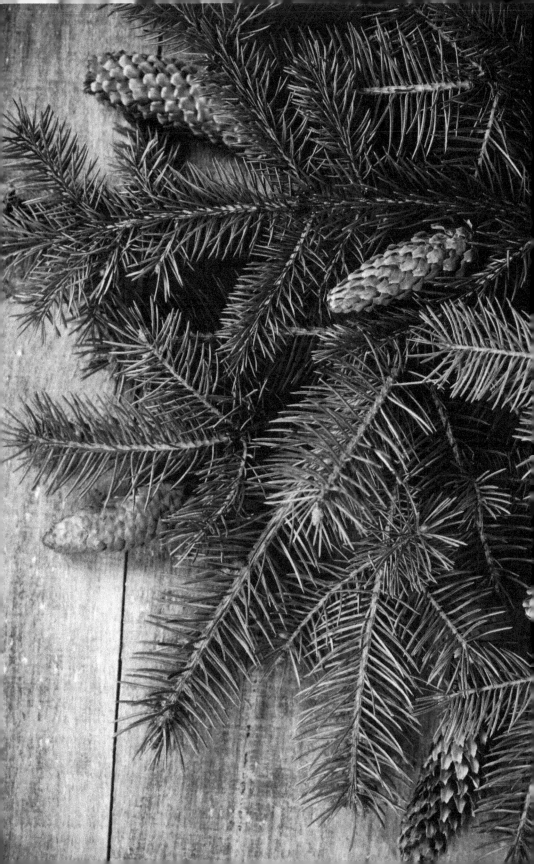

- In a bath
- In a massage oil blend
- In a vaporizer or diffuser

COMPLEMENTARY OILS

- Cedarwood
- Citronella
- Clary sage
- Cypress
- Eucalyptus
- Frankincense
- Lavandin
- Lavender
- Niaouli
- Rosemary
- Sage
- Thyme

WHAT TO WATCH OUT FOR

In large doses, and based on the variety of pine from which it was distilled, pine oil may irritate the skin.

May cause skin irritation

Rose *Rosa damascena*

Rose essential oil may come from a number of different rose varieties. The first distillation of rose essential oil apparently took place in the early 11th century, when the Persian physician Avicenna recorded his use of roses in his medical practice. Rose essential oil is produced from the plant's fresh flowers through steam distillation.

WHAT IT'S USED FOR

- Anger
- Asthma
- Cardiac issues
- Conjunctivitis
- Coughs
- Depression
- Grief
- Hay fever
- High blood pressure
- Liver issues
- Menstrual issues
- Nausea

- Stress
- Tension

HOW IT'S USED

- In a bath
- In a cream blend or lotion blend

- Women's reproductive issues

- In a massage oil blend
- In a vaporizer or diffuser

COMPLEMENTARY OILS

- Bay
- Benzoin
- Clove
- Cedarwood
- Chamomile (German)
- Chamomile (Roman)
- Fennel

- Geranium
- Ginger
- Jasmine
- Lemon
- Melissa
- Palma rosa
- Sandalwood

WHAT TO WATCH OUT FOR

Because it can stimulate menstrual flow, pregnant women should avoid rose oil.

Do not use during pregnancy

Rose Geranium *Pelargonium graveolens*

The rose geranium, native to South Africa, Madagascar, and the Middle East, found its way to southern Europe in the 17th century. Of the plant's 700 varieties, only 10 provide essential oil through steam distillation of the leaves and stalks. The oil's scent combines the fragrance of a rose with notes of mint.

WHAT IT'S USED FOR

- Anxiety
- Burns

- Depression
- Head lice

- Hormonal imbalance
- Oily skin
- Urine retention
- Wounds

- As a shampoo
- In a bath
- In a cream blend or lotion blend
- In a massage oil blend
- In a vaporizer or diffuser

COMPLEMENTARY OILS

- Basil
- Bergamot
- Carrot seed
- Cedarwood
- Citronella
- Clary sage
- Grapefruit
- Jasmine
- Lavender
- Lime
- Neroli
- Orange
- Rosemary

WHAT TO WATCH OUT FOR

Rose geranium oil can irritate the skin. Because of its hormone-balancing properties, pregnant women should avoid rose geranium oil.

Do not use during pregnancy

May cause skin irritation

Rosemary *Rosmarinus officinalis, R. coronarium*

Rosemary essential oil, strongly herbal and stimulating, comes from an evergreen shrub native to Asia and now cultivated in France, Tunisia, and the Slavic countries. Many ancient cultures considered rosemary sacred and used it to ward off evil. The oil is produced from the shrub's flowers through steam distillation.

- Arthritis
- Circulatory issues
- Gout
- Intestinal issues
- Mental fatigue
- Migraine and other types of headaches
- Muscle pain
- Respiratory issues
- Skin puffiness and swelling
- Varicose veins

HOW IT'S USED

- As a shampoo
- In a bath
- In a cream blend or lotion blend
- In a massage oil blend
- In a vaporizer or diffuser

COMPLEMENTARY OILS

- Bay
- Bergamot
- Cassia
- Cedarwood
- Cinnamon
- Citronella
- Cypress
- Geranium
- Hyssop
- Lavandin
- Lavender
- Lemongrass
- Neroli
- Nutmeg
- Palma rosa
- Peppermint
- Pine
- Rose geranium
- Sage
- Spearmint
- Thyme

WHAT TO WATCH OUT FOR

Pregnant women, people with epilepsy, and people with high blood pressure should avoid rosemary oil.

Do not use during pregnancy

Do not use if you have epilepsy

Do not use if you have high blood pressure

Rosewood *Aniba rosaeodora*

An evergreen tree native to the Brazilian rain forest is the source of this floral, spicy oil produced from wood chips through steam distillation. The wood is also used in the construction of cabinets and decorative materials.

WHAT IT'S USED FOR

- Aging skin
- Colds and coughs
- Diminished libido
- Fever
- Headaches
- Immunosuppression

HOW IT'S USED

- In a bath
- In a cream blend or lotion blend
- In a massage oil blend
- In a vaporizer or diffuser

COMPLEMENTARY OILS

- Aniseed
- Bergamot
- Bitter orange
- Grapefruit
- Helichrysum
- Lemon
- Lime
- Orange
- Petitgrain
- Tangerine/mandarin
- Tea tree

WHAT TO WATCH OUT FOR

Rosewood oil may irritate the skin. Do not use rosewood oil around your eyes.

Avoid contact with eyes

May cause skin irritation

Sage *Salvia officinalis*

The medicinal history of this strong and versatile herb goes all the way back to ancient Rome. Sage varieties grow throughout North America as well as in Europe and Asia. The essential oil is produced from the plant's dried leaves through steam distillation. The dried leaves also serve as a popular spice in all kinds of cuisines.

WHAT IT'S USED FOR

- Depression
- Dermatitis
- Digestive issues
- Grief
- Menopausal symptoms
- Menstrual issues
- Skin ulcers
- Stiff neck
- Women's reproductive issues
- Wounds

HOW IT'S USED

- In a bath
- In a cream blend or lotion blend
- In a massage oil blend
- In a vaporizer

COMPLEMENTARY OILS

- Bergamot
- Black pepper
- Lavender
- Lemon
- Pine
- Rosemary

WHAT TO WATCH OUT FOR

Sage oil is toxic when taken internally in large doses. Pregnant women, people with epilepsy, and people with high blood pressure should avoid sage oil. Sage oil should be used very sparingly in aromatherapy.

Do not use during pregnancy

Do not use if you have epilepsy

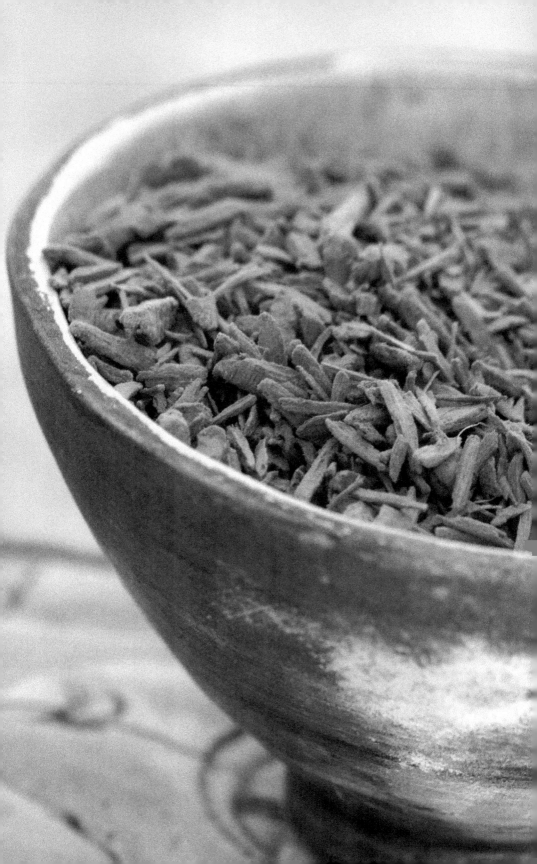

Do not use if you have high blood pressure

May be toxic if taken internally

Sandalwood   *Santalum album*

The beneficent aura of the sandalwood tree belies the tree's parasitic character: to survive, this evergreen extends its roots into other trees and feeds on their nutrients. The tree's wood was used as a building material for millennia, but the sandalwood tree is nearing extinction, and sandalwood essential oil is now the only commercial sandalwood product. To extend the oil's availability, producers create blends of sandalwood with several other essential oils. Look for East Indian sandalwood oil when you want the real thing.

WHAT IT'S USED FOR

- Aging skin
- Bronchial congestion
- Depression
- Itching and inflammation
- Stress
- Tension
- Urinary tract issues

HOW IT'S USED

- In a bath
- In a cream blend or lotion blend
- In a massage oil blend
- In a vaporizer or diffuser

COMPLEMENTARY OILS

- Benzoin
- Bergamot
- Black pepper
- Clary sage
- Clove
- Cypress
- Fennel
- Frankincense
- Geranium
- Ginger
- Jasmine
- Lavender
- Lemon
- Myrrh
- Neroli
- Orange

- Petitgrain
- Rose
- Vetiver
- Ylang-ylang

Sandalwood oil is not associated with any specific warnings.

Spearmint   *Mentha spicata, M. viridis*

A tad sweeter to the nose than peppermint, and safer for use with children, spearmint comes from the Mediterranean region. Spearmint oil is produced from the plant's flowers through steam distillation.

WHAT IT'S USED FOR

- Digestive issues
- Fatigue
- Itching
- Migraine and other types of headaches
- Respiratory issues
- Skin issues
- Stress
- Urine retention

HOW IT'S USED

- In a bath
- In a cream blend or lotion blend
- In a massage oil blend
- In a vaporizer or diffuser

COMPLEMENTARY OILS

- Basil
- Eucalyptus
- Jasmine
- Lavender
- Rosemary

WHAT TO WATCH OUT FOR

Spearmint oil is not associated with any specific warnings.

Spikenard *Nardostachys jatamansi*

The heavy, heady aroma of spikenard comes from a root found in the mountains of northern India as well as in China and Japan. You'll find references to it in the Bible, specifically concerning its use to anoint the feet of Jesus.

WHAT IT'S USED FOR

- Aging skin
- Insomnia
- Migraine
- Stress
- Tension

HOW IT'S USED

- In a bath
- In a massage oil blend
- In a vaporizer

COMPLEMENTARY OILS

- Clary sage
- Lavender
- Lemon
- Neroli
- Patchouli
- Vetiver

WHAT TO WATCH OUT FOR

Spikenard oil is not associated with any specific warnings.

Tagetes *Tagetes minuta, T. glandulifera*

Popularly known as *marigold oil*, tagetes (pronounced *tah-JEE-teez*) is an oil with a sweet, citrusy scent. Although the marigold is native to Africa, where it is gathered in bunches to ward off flies and mosquitoes, it has become a familiar sight in North America gardens. The oil is extracted from the plant's flowers, leaves, and stalks.

- Fungal and parasitic infections
- Respiratory illnesses
- Wounds

HOW IT'S USED

- In a bath
- In a cream blend or lotion blend
- In a massage oil blend
- In a vaporizer or diffuser

COMPLEMENTARY OILS

- Clary sage
- Jasmine
- Lavender
- Lemon
- Myrrh
- Tangerine/mandarin

WHAT TO WATCH OUT FOR

Use tagetes oil sparingly. Tagetes is a photosensitizing oil, so don't use it if you expect to be out in the sun within 12 hours of application, and never add tagetes oil to a tanning or sunscreen blend. Pregnant women should avoid tagetes oil.

Avoid exposure to sunlight for 12 hours after use

Do not use during pregnancy

May cause skin irritation

Tangerine

Citrus reticulata, C. nobilis, C. madurensis, C. unshiu, C. deliciosa

Also known as *true mandarin* and *European mandarin*, this sweet-smelling citrus oil is originally from China, but now the United States is its largest producer. Whether you choose tangerine oil (from fruit harvested in November) or mandarin oil (from the same fruit, but left on the tree until February), you will find the same properties, although mandarin oil has a more pronounced yellow color. The oil can be obtained either through cold-pressing of the rind or through steam distillation of the whole ripe fruit.

WHAT IT'S USED FOR

- Aging skin
- Digestive issues

HOW IT'S USED

- In a bath
- In a cream blend or lotion blend
- In a massage oil blend
- In a vaporizer or diffuser

COMPLEMENTARY OILS

- Aniseed
- Bergamot
- Black pepper
- Carrot seed
- Cinnamon
- Clary sage
- Clove
- Cypress
- Dill
- Frankincense
- Ginger
- Helichrysum
- Hyssop
- Jasmine
- Lavender
- Neroli
- Nutmeg
- Rosewood
- Tagetes

WHAT TO WATCH OUT FOR

Tangerine (mandarin) oil obtained through cold-pressing is a photosensitizing oil, so don't use it if you expect to be out in the sun within 12 hours of application, and never add tangerine (mandarin) oil to a tanning or sunscreen blend. Oils obtained by cold-pressing don't last long, so they need to be used within six months.

Avoid exposure to sunlight for 12 hours after use

May cause skin irritation

Use within six months of purchase date

Tea Tree *Melaleuca alternifolia*

Tea tree oil comes from a type of small tree that grows in the Australian state of New South Wales. You may see bottles of it labeled *ti-trol* or *melasol*, so check for the botanical name to be sure of what you have. Tea tree oil, found in pharmacies, spas, and salons around the world, is one of the most popular and widely used essential oils. It is produced from the tea tree's leaves and twigs through steam distillation.

WHAT IT'S USED FOR

- Dandruff
- Infections
- Respiratory issues
- Sunburn
- Wounds

HOW IT'S USED

- As a wash
- In a bath
- In a cream blend or lotion blend
- In a massage oil blend
- In a vaporizer or diffuser
- In neat (undiluted) applications

COMPLEMENTARY OILS

- Chamomile (German)
- Cinnamon
- Clary sage
- Clove
- Geranium
- Lavender
- Lemon
- Lemongrass
- Marjoram
- Myrrh
- Nutmeg
- Rosemary
- Rosewood
- Thyme

WHAT TO WATCH OUT FOR

Tea tree oil may irritate the skin. Do not use tea tree oil on deep wounds. Do not use tea tree oil around your eyes or mucous membranes. Do not take tea tree oil internally.

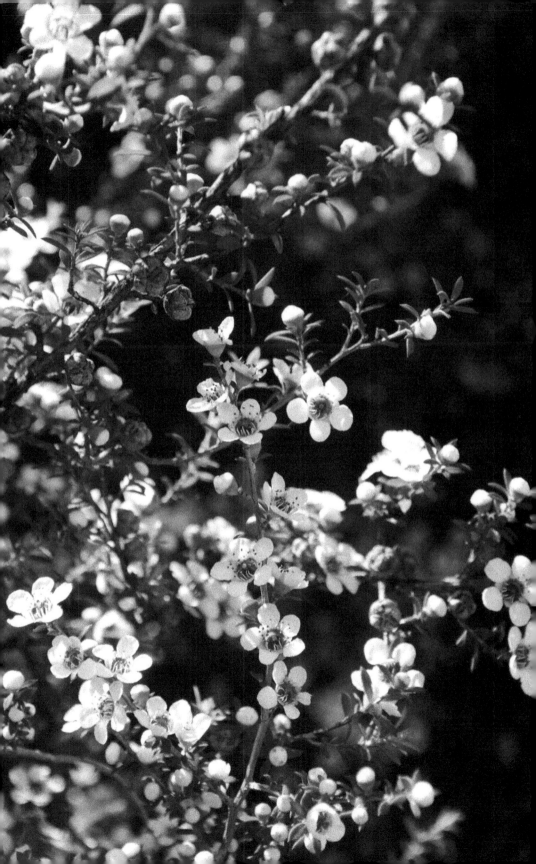

Avoid contact with eyes

Avoid contact with mucous membranes

May be toxic if taken internally

May cause skin irritation

Thyme *Thymus vulgaris, T. aestivus, T. ilerdensis, T. velantianus*

Strangely sweet, given its herbal origins, thyme oil comes from one of the primary plants used in ancient medical practices. The oil is produced from the herb's flowering tops and leaves through steam distillation.

WHAT IT'S USED FOR

- Animal bites
- Arthritis
- Gout
- Respiratory issues
- Sciatica

HOW IT'S USED

- In a massage oil blend
- In a vaporizer or diffuser
- In neat (undiluted) applications (animal bites only)

COMPLEMENTARY OILS

- Bay
- Bergamot
- Cajeput
- Cinnamon
- Eucalyptus
- Grapefruit
- Lavandin
- Lavender
- Lemon
- Pine
- Rosemary
- Tea tree

WHAT TO WATCH OUT FOR

Do not use thyme oil if you have high blood pressure. Because it can speed up the birth process and aid in expulsion of the placenta, pregnant women who are not in labor should avoid thyme oil.

Do not use during pregnancy

Do not use if you have high blood pressure

Vetiver *Vetiveria zizanioides, Andropogon muricatus*

This oil, with its delightfully musty scent, comes from a tropical grass native to India, Tahiti, Java, and Haiti. The oil is produced from the plant's roots through steam distillation.

WHAT IT'S USED FOR

- Anger
- Arthritis
- Exhaustion
- Insomnia
- Muscle aches
- Stress

HOW IT'S USED

- In a bath
- In a cream blend or lotion blend
- In a massage oil blend
- In a vaporizer or diffuser

COMPLEMENTARY OILS

- Benzoin
- Bergamot
- Grapefruit
- Jasmine
- Juniper berry
- Lavender
- Orange
- Sandalwood
- Spikenard
- Ylang-ylang

WHAT TO WATCH OUT FOR

Vetiver is not associated with any specific warnings.

Ylang-Ylang   *Cananga odorata, Unona odorantissimum*

One of the most exotic sweet oils, ylang-ylang comes from a tree native to Java, Sumatra, the island of Réunion, the Comoro Islands, and Madagascar. If you're old enough to recall the macassar oils that men once used in their hair—and the antimacassars that our grand-mothers and great-grandmothers placed on the arms and backs of upholstered chairs to protect them from this oil—then you may remember the scent of ylang-ylang. The first distillation of this oil comes from the tree's fresh flowers, and afterward some distillers make an absolute and a concrete (see page 12 for more about abso-lute and concrete in solvent extraction).

WHAT IT'S USED FOR

- Anxiety
- Diminished libido
- Dry skin
- High blood pressure
- Scalp issues
- Stress
- Tension

HOW IT'S USED

- In a cream blend or lotion blend
- In a massage oil blend
- In a vaporizer or diffuser

COMPLEMENTARY OILS

- Allspice
- Bay
- Bergamot
- Black pepper
- Chamomile (German)
- Grapefruit
- Ginger
- Lavender
- Lime
- Melissa
- Neroli
- Palma rosa
- Sandalwood
- Vetiver

Excessive use of ylang-ylang oil can cause headaches and nausea. Ylang-ylang oil can irritate the skin.

May cause skin irritation

May cause headache

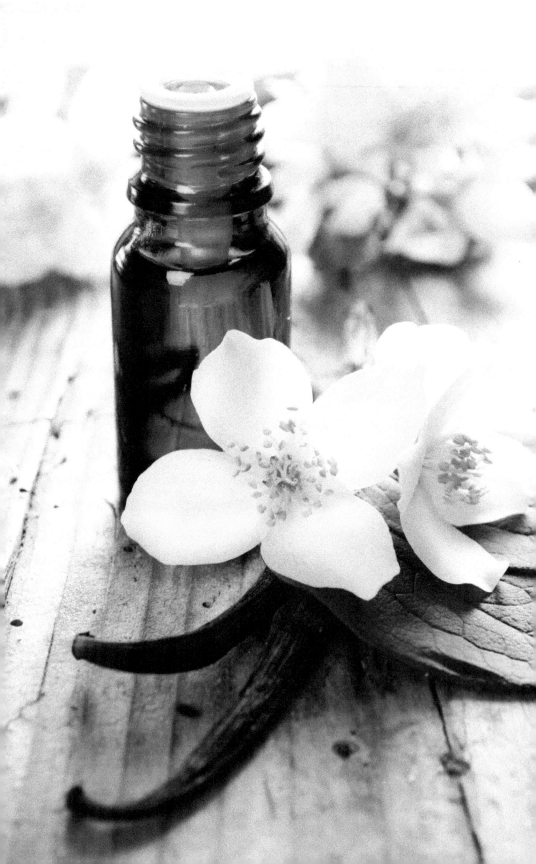

TOP 25 ESSENTIAL OILS AND HOW TO USE THEM

ANALGESIC

Basil 232

Bergamot 236

Black pepper 238

Chamomile
   (German) 245

Chamomile
   (Roman) 246

Eucalyptus 256

Geranium 260

Ginger 262

Juniper berry 269

Lavender 271

Peppermint 288

Rosemary 294

Tea tree 304

ANTIDEPRESSANT

Basil 232

Bergamot 236

Clary sage 250

Geranium 260

Jasmine 268

Lavender 271

Lemon 272

Orange 285

Patchouli 287

Rosemary 294

Ylang-ylang 308

ANTIFUNGAL AGENT

Basil 232

Chamomile
   (German) 245

Clary sage 250

Geranium 260

Helichrysum 265

Patchouli 287

Peppermint 288

Rosemary 294

Tea tree 304

ANTI-INFLAMMATORY

Basil 232

Chamomile
   (German) 245

Geranium 260

Helichrysum 265

Lavender 271

Patchouli 287

Peppermint 288

Rosemary 294

Tea tree 304

ANTI-SCARRING AGENT

Bergamot 236

Chamomile
   (German) 245

Eucalyptus 256

Frankincense 259

Geranium 260

Helichrysum 265

Lavender 271

Lemon 272

Patchouli 287

Rosemary 294

Tea tree 304

Thyme 306

ANTISEPTIC

Basil 232

Bergamot 236

Black pepper 238

Cedarwood 244

Chamomile
   (Roman) 246

Cinnamon 248

Cypress 254

Frankincense 259

Geranium 260

Ginger 262

Helichrysum 265

Jasmine 268

Juniper berry 269

Lavender 271

Lemon 272

Patchouli 287

Peppermint 288

Rosemary 294

Tea tree 304

Thyme 306

Ylang-ylang 308

ANTISPASMODIC

Basil 232
Black pepper 238
Chamomile
    (German) 245
Chamomile
    (Roman) 246
Cinnamon 248
Clary sage 250
Cypress 254
Eucalyptus 256
Geranium 260
Helichrysum 265
Jasmine 268
Juniper berry 269
Lavender 271
Lemon 272
Orange 285
Peppermint 288
Thyme 306

APHRODISIAC

Cinnamon 248
Jasmine 268
Patchouli 287
Rosemary 294
Ylang-ylang 308

ASTRINGENT

Cedarwood 244
Cypress 254
Eucalyptus 256
Frankincense 259
Geranium 260
Juniper berry 269
Lemon 272
Patchouli 287
Peppermint 288
Rosemary 294

CALMING AGENT

Basil 232
Clary sage 250
Geranium 260
Juniper berry 269
Lavender 271
Lemon 272

CARMINATIVE

Basil 232
Bergamot 236
Black pepper 238
Chamomile
    (German) 245
Chamomile
    (Roman) 246
Cinnamon 248
Frankincense 259
Ginger 262
Juniper berry 269
Lavender 271
Lemon 272
Orange 285
Peppermint 288
Rosemary 294
Thyme 306

CEPHALIC AGENT

Basil 232
Peppermint 288
Rosemary 294

DECONGESTANT

Chamomile
    (German) 245
Clary sage 250
Eucalyptus 256
Geranium 260
Juniper berry 269
Lavender 271
Lemon 272
Orange 285
Patchouli 287
Peppermint 288
Rosemary 294

DEODORANT

Bergamot 236
Clary sage 250
Cypress 254
Eucalyptus 256
Geranium 260
Lavender 271
Patchouli 287

DIGESTIVE

Basil 232
Chamomile
    (German) 245
Chamomile
    (Roman) 246
Geranium 260
Helichrysum 265
Orange 285
Peppermint 288
Rosemary 294

DISINFECTANT

Bergamot 236
Eucalyptus 256
Geranium 260
Helichrysum 265
Lavender 271
Lemon 272
Patchouli 287
Rosemary 294
Tea tree 304
Thyme 306

DIURETIC

Cedarwood 244
Cypress 254
Eucalyptus 256
Frankincense 259
Geranium 260
Helichrysum 265
Lavender 271
Patchouli 287
Rosemary 294
Thyme 306

EXPECTORANT

Basil 232
Cedarwood 244
Eucalyptus 256
Frankincense 259
Ginger 262
Helichrysum 265
Peppermint 288
Tea tree 304
Thyme 306

FEBRIFUGE

Basil 232
Bergamot 236
Black pepper 238
Eucalyptus 256
Ginger 262
Lemon 272
Patchouli 287
Peppermint 288

HORMONE INFLUENCERS

Basil 232
Chamomile
  (German) 245
Chamomile
  (Roman) 246
Clary sage 250
Geranium 260
Helichrysum 265
Peppermint 288
Rosemary 294
Ylang-ylang 308

IMMUNE SYSTEM BOOSTER

Cypress 254
Frankincense 259
Patchouli 287
Tea tree 304

RUBEFACIENT

Eucalyptus 256
Ginger 262
Juniper berry 269
Lemon 272
Rosemary 294

SEDATIVE

Bergamot 236
Cedarwood 244
Chamomile
  (German) 245
Chamomile
  (Roman) 246
Clary sage 250
Frankincense 259
Jasmine 268
Lavender 271
Orange 285
Patchouli 287
Ylang-ylang 308

STIMULANT

Basil 232
Cinnamon 248
Ginger 262
Juniper berry 269
Peppermint 288
Rosemary 294
Tea tree 304
Thyme 306

TONIC

Basil 232
Bergamot 236
Black pepper 238
Clary sage 250
Cypress 254
Ginger 262
Helichrysum 265
Juniper berry 269
Lemon 272
Rosemary 294
Thyme 306

VULNERARY

Bergamot 236
Chamomile
  (German) 245
Chamomile
  (Roman) 246
Eucalyptus 256
Frankincense 259
Geranium 260
Juniper berry 269
Lavender 271

KNOW YOUR BRANDS

AURA CACIA

Where to buy Aura Cacia products: At wellness centers, health food stores, some drugstores, and AuraCacia.com

Price range: Half-ounce bottles (one-third of an ounce for the organic line) priced lower than some products from other makers

About the company: Independently tests oils it receives from its sources to ensure products' purity; lists all ingredients on bottles; goal is to "make aromatherapy easy"

Reviews: Very favorable, reflecting a reputation for product purity and effectiveness

DŌTERRA

Where to buy dōTerra products: At house parties, from a "consultant" (this is an MLM arrangement), or online at doTerra.com

Price range: High (discounts for "consultants")

About the company: Newcomer (2008) to MLM category; sells single essential oils and blends; registered trademark "Certified Pure Therapeutic Grade" reflects company standards; limited selection of oils and blends

Reviews: Very favorable overall

ESOTERIC OILS

Where to buy Esoteric Oils products: Online at Essential Oils.co.za

Price range: Moderate to high; products include 11-milliliter bottles of essential oils as well as 110-milliliter bottles of special blends

About the company: Esoteric Oils sells 100 percent pure and unadulterated essential oils, as well as pre-blended treatment oils. The essential oils are extracted from renewable resources grown on smaller family-based farms that do not rely on chemical fertilizers and pesticides. The company is based in South Africa and uses fair-trade practices in purchasing plant materials to make its oils.

Reviews: Very favorable

ESSENTIAL VITALITY

Where to buy Essential Vitality products: Online at QueensHome Schooling.com

Price range: Moderate; oils packaged in distinctive 5-milliliter cobalt bottles, smaller than those of some other providers but more affordable

About the company: Rebrands oils purchased from a variety of distillers and that are made from plants grown organically, without the use of pesticides; started by practitioners at the Holistic Wellness Center in New Freeport, Pennsylvania; researched and selected the oils to be used in their proprietary blends

Reviews: Generally favorable, but scarce because this company's distribution is limited

HERITAGE ESSENTIAL OILS

Where to buy Heritage Essential Oils products: Online at HeritageEssentialOils.com or at the company's general store in Waco, Texas

Price range: Moderate; smaller bottles available to fit tighter budgets

About the company: Careful to make no therapeutic claims; organically grown products; 2-milliliter samples available of just about any essential oil

Reviews: Very favorable (and not to be confused with reviews for Heritage Store, another company)

MOUNTAIN ROSE HERBS

Where to buy Mountain Rose Herbs products: Online at MountainRoseHerbs.com

Price range: Moderate

About the company: Sells only 100 percent steam-distilled, undiluted oils except for a few that must be extracted with other methods; also sell teas, herbs, spices, and natural health products

Reviews: Raves, but with a very small company's reputation for somewhat spotty customer service

NATIVE AMERICAN NUTRITIONALS

Where to buy Native American Nutritionals products: Online at NativeAmericanNutritionals.com

Price range: With single oils available in 15-milliliter bottles, less expensive than most brands

About the company: Features interesting essential oil blends, labeled for their expected effects; many already contain a carrier oil, for customers who prefer to buy a blend; also carries single oils and carrier oils

Reviews: Very favorable

NORTH AMERICAN HERB AND SPICE

Where to buy North American Herb and Spice products: At vitamin shops and natural food stores or at online vendors

Price range: Moderate

About the company: In addition to essential oils also sells various items from dietary supplements to cleaning products; essential oils labeled as blends; users have high praise for the healing properties of these blends

Reviews: Very favorable

SCENTASTICS 2

Where to buy Scentastics 2 products: Online at Scentastics2.com or at fairs and festivals

Price range: Low

About the company: Sells 100 percent essential oils as well as perfume and fragrance oils and other scented products; often at fairs, festivals, and crafts shows in New England; an economy supplier; use clear glass bottles that you will want to transfer into amber bottles

Reviews: None to date

YOUNG LIVING

Where to buy Young Living products: At house parties (MLM) or online at YoungLiving.com

Price range: Highest (lower prices for the company's "wholesale members")

About the company: Owns the trademark to the phrases "The World Leader in Essential Oils," and "Young Living Therapeutic Grade"; similar to dōTerra, claims that the nonexistent "therapeutic grade" designation refers to internal quality standards; maintains it's own supply chain, able to regulate the growing, production, bottling, labeling, and sale of its products

Reviews: Favorable

GLOSSARY

absolute: An alcohol-based essential oil extract with 5 to 10 parts per million of solvent residue remaining from the extraction process.

adulterated: An oil that contains anything but pure, 100 percent essential oil.

analgesic: A substance that relieves pain.

aphrodisiac: A substance that promotes sexual desire.

aromatherapy: The use of scent for medicinal or mental health benefits.

astringent: A substance that contracts body tissues, reducing discharges like oils.

bulking: Using plants from the same species but from different harvests to bring down the cost of a specific oil.

carminative: A substance that prevents gas from forming in the intestinal tract.

carrier oil: An oil used to dilute essential oils, literally carrying the essential oil to the skin. Most essential oils need to be diluted in a carrier oil before being applied to skin to reduce the risk of irritation.

cephalic: A substance that has the ability to clear the head (for clarity of thought).

chain of supply: The number of companies involved in the process to get the plants in the field to your home in the form of essential oils. This can include the growers, distillers, processors, bottlers, distributors, retailers, therapists, and personal sales consultants who have an influence on the product before you buy it.

cicatrizant: A substance that promotes healing through the formation of scar tissue.

cold-pressing: See *expression*.

concrete: A substance that includes the terpenes, chlorophyll, plant tissue, and fats or waxes contained in the plant.

constituent: The part of an oil that gives it its therapeutic value.

diffuser: A device that is used to release the scent of an essential oil or blend into the air.

dilutant: A colorless, odorless synthetic additive that allows bottlers to stretch the supply of an essential oil by diluting it.

distillation: Using steam and/or water to break down a plant's leaves, stems, flowers, roots, or bark.

diuretic: A substance that encourages the production of urine.

double-blind: A study in which some information is concealed from the tester and the subject to prevent bias in the results. Studies in which one group receives a test drug and another receives a placebo are double-blind when neither the researcher nor the subject knows who received which substance.

drop: A measure of 1/600 of a fluid ounce of oil.

essential oil: A liquid extracted from plant material that contains the essence of the plant's scent.

expectorant: A substance that encourages phlegm and congestion to break up.

expression: Using a mechanical process to rotate and puncture the rind of fruit to collect the juice and essential oil released from the rind.

extender: A chemical additive that contains fragrance.

febrifuge: A substance that aids in lowering fever.

fixed oil: A natural oil that does not change its state when heated.

fragrance oil: An oil that includes chemicals or blends of synthetics, and that is used most commonly as a perfume or air freshener.

humidifier: A device that creates warm or cool mist to keep the air in a room moist.

hypercritical carbon dioxide (CO_2) extraction: Using very high pressure to take gaseous carbon dioxide to a point at which the physical line between liquid and gas dissolves. This creates a dense liquid that can pass through plant material, extracting specific compounds.

in vitro: Research conducted in a laboratory, usually using cells or tissue, but not using animal or human subjects.

in vivo: Research conducted on living subjects.

maceration: Using hot oil to rupture a plant's cell membranes and extract the plant's essence.

nature identical oil: A synthetic product that may contain extenders, dilutants, or other additives.

nebulizer: A device that is used to deliver medication directly into the lungs and bronchial system using compressed air.

perfume oil: A fragrance made primarily from synthetic compounds.

photosensitization: The ability of some plants to make your skin more susceptible to damage from the ultraviolet rays of the sun.

pipette: A glass tube that allows you to measure and transfer tiny amounts of essential oils.

placebo: A pill or other simulated medical treatment that contains no medicinal compounds.

pure: An oil that has no ingredients except for 100 percent essential oil.

rubefacient: A substance that brings rosy color to the face.

solvent extraction: Using a solvent (methanol, ethanol, hexane, or petroleum ether) to pull the scented molecules out of a plant.

terpene: An organic compound produced by a plant to create an aroma. Terpenes are the main component in an essential oil.

therapeutic grade: A term made up by some manufacturers and distributors in the essential oil industry. There is no such thing as an official "therapeutic grade," as the essential oil industry is not regulated by the federal government.

topical: A substance that is used on the outside of the body.

vaporizer: A device that creates steam to keep the air in a room moist.

volatile organic compounds (VOCs): Naturally occurring chemicals that have a low boiling point and a high vapor pressure at room temperature. Most scents are made of VOCs.

vulnerary: A substance that is useful in healing wounds.

ADDITIONAL READING

Anisman-Reiner, Victoria. "Natural Psoriasis Treatments Using Essential Oils." Suite.io. September 10, 2009. https://suite.io/victoria-anisman-reiner/2802280.

——. "Natural Ringworm Treatment Using Essential Oils." Suite.io. September 11, 2009. https://suite.io/victoria-anisman-reiner/285j280.

Apter, Joan. "Article 2: The History of Essential Oils." Joan Apter Aromatherapy. Accessed June 5, 2014. www.apteraromatherapy.com/articles2.html.

AromaWeb. "Aromatherapy Recipes to Enhance Memory and Concentration." Accessed June 20, 2014. www.aromaweb.com/recipes/memory.asp.

——. "Guide to Diluting Essential Oils." Accessed June 15, 2014. www.aromaweb.com/articles/dilutingessentialoils.asp.

——. "How to Buy Essential Oils." Accessed June 7, 2014. www.aromaweb.com/articles/howtobuyessentialoils.asp.

——. "Storing Essential Oils." Accessed June 9, 2014. www.aromaweb.com/articles/storing.asp.

Aura Cacia. "For the Home." Accessed June 27, 2014. www.auracacia.com/store.php?Screen=recipes&collection=forthehome&dsp=collection.

——. "Green Cleaning with Essential Oils." Accessed June 26, 2014. www.auracacia.com/auracacia/aclearn/art_greenclean.html.

Baby Steps to Essential Oils (blog). "Indigestion and Reflux Remedies with Young Living Essential Oils." July 2, 2013. http://babystepstoessentialoils.com/2013/07/02/indigestion-reflux-remedies-with-young-living-essential-oils/.

Banks, Suzanne R. "Help Your Hangover with Essential Oils." suzannerbanks (blog). March 4, 2013. http://suzannerbanks.wordpress.com/2013/03/04/help-your-hangover-with-essential-oils/.

The Base Formula (blog). "Essential Oils That Your Liver Will Love!" January 24, 2012. www.baseformula.com/blog/2012/01/essential-oils-that-your-liver-will-love/.

Boice, Melissa. "Emotional Relief with Essential Oils." *Neat Oil Essentials* (blog). Accessed June 24, 2014. http://neatoilessentials.com/emotional-relief -essential-oils/.

Cooksley, Valerie. "Can Essential Oils Help with Hair Loss?" *Natural Health Magazine.* Accessed June 23, 2014. www.naturalhealthmag.com/expert-advice /can-essential-oils-help-hair-loss.

Crunchy Betty. "3+ Ways to Naturally Dissolve Cellulite without Breaking a Sweat." *Crunchy Betty* (blog). September 21, 2010. www.crunchybetty .com/3-ways-to-naturally-dissolve-cellulite-without-breaking-a-sweat.

dōTerra. "Uses of Essential Oils." Accessed June 16, 2014. www.mydoterra.com /kimlayton/essentialUses.html.

dōTerra Blog. "DIY: Deodorant Stick." January 4, 2014. http://doterrablog.com /diy-deodorant-stick/.

Esoteric Oils. "Blisters." Accessed June 19, 2014. www.essentialoils.co.za /treatment/blisters.htm.

———. "Compresses." Accessed June 16, 2014. www.essentialoils.co.za /compresses.htm.

———. "Halitosis (Bad Breath)." Accessed June 22, 2014. www.essentialoils .co.za/treatment/halitosis.htm.

———. "The History of Essential Oils and Aromatherapy." Accessed June 2, 2014. www.essentialoils.co.za/history-essential-oils.htm.

Evans, Linsay. "Home Remedies for Chafed Skin." azcentral.com. Accessed June 19, 2014. http://healthyliving.azcentral.com/home-remedies-chafed-skin -1853.html.

EverythingEssential.me. "A Brief History of Essential Oils." Accessed June 2, 2014. www.everythingessential.me/AboutOils/History.html.

———. "Colic." Accessed June 20, 2014. www.everythingessential.me /HealthConcerns/Colic.html#page=page-2.

———. "Hemorrhoids." Accessed June 23, 2014. www.everythingessential.me /HealthConcerns/Hemorrhoids.html#page=page-2.

———. "Liver Disease (Hepatic Disease)." Accessed June 23, 2014. www .everythingessential.me/HealthConcerns/LiverDisease.html#page=page-2.

Experience-Essential-Oils.com. "Looking for a Natural Muscle Relaxer for Spasms and Overexerted Muscles? Use Essential Oils!" Accessed June 23, 2014. www.experience-essential-oils.com/natural-muscle-relaxer.html.

——. "Natural Remedy for Nausea and Vomiting—Essential Oils Are the Perfect Solution." Accessed June 20, 2014. www.experience-essential-oils.com /natural-remedy-for-nausea.html.

——. "Spider Bite Remedies Are Made Easy with Essential Oils." Accessed June 18, 2014. www.experience-essential-oils.com/spider-bite-remedies.html.

Gaia Life Oils (blog). "Underestimated Peppermint!" October 16, 2011. http://gaialifeoils.com/tag/flatulence/.

Gallagher, Jen. "Essential Oil and Herbs for Gourmet Cooking." Essential Oil Goddess. Accessed June 16, 2014. www.essential-oil-goddess.com/essential-oil -and-herbs.html.

Green, Nastassia. "Almond Oil vs. Sweet Almond Oil: How to Choose the Best Almond Oil." Oilpedia. Accessed July 8, 2014. http://oilypedia.com /almond-oil-vs-sweet-almond-oil-how-to-choose-the-best-almond-oil/.

Guba, Ron. "The Modern Alchemy of Carbon Dioxide Extraction." *International Journal of Aromatherapy* 12, no. 3 (2002): 120–6. www.scribd.com /doc/7574112/The-Modern-Alchemy-of-Carbon-Dioxide-Extraction.

Heritage Essential Oils. "Skin Tag." Accessed June 24, 2014. http:// heritageessentialoils.com/skin-tag.php.

Hobbs, Christopher. "Understanding Essential Oils." In *Herbal Remedies for Dummies* (New York: Wiley Publishing, 1998). www.dummies.com/how-to /content/understanding-essential-oils.html.

Holland, Stephanie. "Top 3 Essential Oils to Reduce High Blood Pressure." Suite.io. October 31, 2010. https://suite.io/stephanie-holland/4dqd21q.

Home Remedy Shop. "9 Home Remedies to Get Rid of Ingrown Toenail." November 20, 2013. www.homeremedyshop.com/9-home-remedies-to -get-rid-of-ingrown-toenail/.

Homestead, Carol. "Essential Oil Combinations for Anti Aging." *LifeCell Anti Aging Tips* (blog). January 10, 2014. www.lifecellantiagingtips.com /essential-oil-combinations-use-skin/.

Ishum, Rebecca. "Essential Oils: The German, British, and French Schools of Thought." *A Beautiful Ruckus* (blog). May 4, 2014. www.abeautifulruckus .com/2014/05/essential-oils-german-british-and.html.

Johnson, S., and K. Boren. "Topical and Oral Administration of Essential Oils— Safety Issues." *Aromatopia* 22, no. 4 (July 2013): 43–8. http://yoursacredcalling .com/commonscentsmom/wp-content/uploads/2012/06/internal-ingestion -document.pdf.

Keniston-Pond, Kymberly. "Essential Oils for Seasonal Allergy Relief." Richmond Natural Medicine. Accessed June 18, 2014. http://richmondnaturalmed.com/essential-oils-for-seasonal-allergy-relief/.

Kepes, Carolyn. "Essential Oils for Enhancing Energy." Living Naturally. Accessed June 22, 2014. www.livingnaturally.com/PDFDocs/n /NP7SQHE2NLQS9J0XD5APLFXRS0925MR2.PDF.

Kitchen Stewardship (blog). "It's Scary When Your Child Can't Breathe (Natural Remedies for Croup)." April 1, 2013. www.kitchenstewardship.com/2013/04/01 /its-scary-when-your-child-cant-breathe-natural-remedies-for-croup/.

Kwitt, Lynn. "Layering vs. Blending Essential Oils." The Joy of Essential Oils. October 30, 2010. http://thejoyofessentialoils.com/2010/10/30 /layering-vs-blending-essential-oils/.

LCL Beauty. "Personal and Home Use Tap Water Aromatherapy Facial Steamer with Ozone." Accessed June 14, 2014. http://lclbeauty.com/proddetail .php?prod=PRO-111.

Liu, J. H., G. H. Chen, H. Z. Yeh, C. K. Huang, and S. K. Poon. "Enteric-Coated Peppermint-Oil Capsules in the Treatment of Irritable Bowel Syndrome: A Prospective, Randomized Trial." *Journal of Gastroenterology* 32, no. 6 (December 1997): 765–8. www.ncbi.nlm.nih.gov/pubmed/9430014.

Lyth, Geoff. "Shelf Life of Aromatherapy Oils." Quinessence Aromatherapy. Accessed June 8, 2014. www.quinessence.com/shelf_life.htm.

———. "Storing Your Essential Oils." Quinessence Aromatherapy. Accessed June 8, 2014. www.quinessence.com/essential_oil_storage_methods.htm.

Meyers, Angela. "doTerra Essential Oil to Treat Acid Reflux and Heartburn Naturally." *Healing Heart Oils* (blog). October 7, 2012. http://healingheartoils .blogspot.com/2012/10/doterra-essential-oil-for-acid-reflux.html.

Mitchell, Marlene. "Aromatherapy and Moods." International Certified Aromatherapy Institute. May 29, 2012. www.aromatherapyinstitute.com /view_article.php?id=42.

Moore, Kristeen. "Humidifiers and Health." Healthline.com. July 18, 2012. www.healthline.com/health/humidifiers-and-health#Overview1.

movableqi (blog). "Young Living Essential Oils and Men's Health & Wellness." June 4, 2012. http://movableqi.wordpress.com/2012/06/04 /young-living-essential-oils-and-mens-health-wellness/.

National Association for Holistic Aromatherapy. "Exploring Aromatherapy: How Are Essential Oils Extracted?" Accessed June 4, 2014. www.naha.org /explore-aromatherapy/about-aromatherapy/how-are-essential-oils -extracted.

———. "Exploring Aromatherapy: Safety Information." Accessed June 16, 2014. www.naha.org/explore-aromatherapy/safety/.

———. "Exploring Aromatherapy: What is Aromatherapy?" Accessed June 5, 2014. www.naha.org/explore-aromatherapy/about-aromatherapy/what-is -aromatherapy.

National Institute of Arthritis and Musculoskeletal and Skin Diseases. "What Is Acne?" National Institutes of Health. Last modified November 2010. www .niams.nih.gov/Health_Info/Acne/acne_ff.asp.

"Natural Treatments for Prostate Enlargement and Prostatitis." Accessed June 24, 2014. www.dcdoctor.com/pages/rightpages_wellnesscenter/naturaltxs/pages /diet_tx_prostate.html#DIET/NUTR-TX-PROSTATE-back%20to%20menu.

Nature's Gift. "Methods of Application." Accessed June 15, 2014. www .naturesgift.com/methods.htm.

Nordqvist, Christian. "What is Aromatherapy? The Theory Behind Aromatherapy." Medical News Today (MNT). July 8, 2009. www .medicalnewstoday.com/articles/10884.php.

Oils and Plants. "Cystitis." Accessed June 22, 2014. www.oilsandplants.com /cystitis.htm.

The Paleo Mama (blog). "Essential Oils for Seasonal Allergies." March 24, 2014. http://thepaleomama.com/2014/03/essential-oils-seasonal-allergies/.

Rozenn, Maureen H. "Essential Oil Therapy." Accessed June 16, 2014. http:// acupuncturesantacruz.net/about-chinese-medicine/essential-oil-therapy/.

Surber, Chelsea. "Aromatherapy vs. Medical Grade Nebulizers." *Just Nebulizers Blog*. November 17, 2009. http://justnebulizers.com/respiratory-blog /aromatherapy-nebulizer/#.U54QARZ7x8s.

Sustainable Baby Steps. "How to Use Essential Oils with Four Applications." Accessed June 15, 2014. www.sustainablebabysteps.com/how-to-use-essential -oils.html.

University of Maryland Medical Center. "Aromatherapy: Overview." Last modified May 7, 2013. http://umm.edu/health/medical/altmed/treatment /aromatherapy.

U.S. Food and Drug Administration. "Essential Oils, Oleoresins (Solvent-Free), and Natural Extractives (Including Distillates)." Section 182.20 in Code of Federal Regulations Title 21, vol. 3. Last modified April 1, 2013. www .accessdata.fda.gov/scripts/cdrh/cfdocs/cfcfr/CFRSearch.cfm?fr=182.20.

WebMD. "First Aid and Emergencies: Brown Recluse Spider Bite Treatment." Accessed June 18, 2014. www.webmd.com/first-aid/spider-bite-brown -recluse-spider-bite-treatment.

Wings and Heroes. "Stopping Hiccups." Accessed June 23, 2014. www .wingsandheros.com/articles/essential-oils/stopping-hiccups.html.

ESSENTIAL OILS AND CARRIER OILS INDEX

* **Boldface** indicates a major discussion.

A
...
Ajowan essential oil, 30
Allspice essential oil, 168, **230**
Aloe vera carrier oil, 28, 179
Ambrette seed essential oil, 168
Amyris essential oil, 168
Angelica essential oil, 35, 36, 162, 164
Anise. *See* Aniseed essential oil
Aniseed essential oil, 33, **230–231**
Antiseed essential oil, 32
Apricot kernel carrier oil, 28, 62, 108, 130, 204
Avocado carrier oil, 28, 61, 72, 108, 110, 120, 183
Azob. *See* Hyssop essential oil

B
...
Balsam fir essential oil, 81, 168
Balsam of Peru essential oil, 30
Basil essential oil, 32, 33, 72, 95, 122, 134, 136, 138, 153, 155, 186, 192, 194, **232–233**, 311, 312
Bastard lavender. *See* Lavandin essential oil
Bay essential oil, 32, 33, **233–234**

Bee balm. *See* Melissa essential oil
Benjamin. *See* Benzoin essential oil
Benzoin essential oil, 34, **234–236**
Bergamot essential oil, 10, 35, 49, 66, 129, 130, 141, 146, 153, 154, 158, 168, 171, 188, 189, 209, 217, **236–238**, 311, 312, 313
Bitter almond essential oil, 30
Bitter orange essential oil, 35, 49, 84
Black pepper essential oil, 84, 97, 153, 168, **238–239**, 311, 312, 313
Blue chamomile. *See* German chamomile essential oil
Blue cypress essential oil, 61, 120
Blue gum. *See* Eucalyptus essential oil
Bois de rose essential oil, 61
Boldo leaf essential oil, 30
Borage seed essential oil, 61, 178
Buchu essential oil, 33

C
...
Cade oil crude essential oil, 30
Cajeput essential oil, **239–241**
Cajuput. *See* Cajeput essential oil

Calamus essential oil, 32
Calendula carrier oil, 28, 192
Calendula essential oil, 80, 98
Camphor essential oil, 30, 32, 33
Caraway essential oil, **241–242**
Cardamom essential oil, 97, 168
Carnation essential oil, 34
Carrot carrier oil, 178
Carrot essential oil, 59, 61, 104
Carrot seed carrier oil, 180
Carrot seed essential oil, 64, 98, 108, 141, **242**
Cassia bark. *See* Cassia essential oil
Cassia essential oil, 33, **243**
Castor carrier oil, 119
Catnip essential oil, 133
Cayenne essential oil, 147
Cedarwood essential oil, 123, 141, 148, 168, 194, 202, **244–245**, 312, 313
Ceylon cinnamon. *See* Cinnamon essential oil
Chamomile essential oil, 34, 36, 59, 66, 73, 74, 75, 99, 109, 127, 142, 153, 154, 164, 176, 192, 202, 212, 217. *See also* German chamomile essential oil; Roman chamomile essential oil

Chinese cinnamon. *See* Cassia essential oil

Chinese parsley. *See* Coriander essential oil

Chocolate peppermint essential oil, 168

Choomana poolu. *See* Lemongrass essential oil

Cinnamon essential oil, 32, 33, 36, 49, 102, 115, 145, 146, 148, 153, 168, 217, 222, **248–249,** 312, 313

Citronella essential oil, 32, 133, 185, **249**

Clary sage essential oil, 36, 58, 66, 72, 133, 141, 143, 145, 158, 160, 162, 164, 202, 209, **250–251,** 311, 312

Clary wort. *See* Clary sage essential oil

Clear eye. *See* Clary sage essential oil

Clove essential oil, 32, 33, 49, 67, 90, 92, 102, 168, 169, 171, 173, 222, **251–253**

Coconut carrier oil, 59, 60, 89, 90, 109, 113, 117, 119, 142, 170, 171, 180, 186, 202, 203, 204, 206, 207, 211

Coriander essential oil, 168, **253–254**

Costusroot essential oil, 30

Croton essential oil, 30

Cumin essential oil, 35

Cypress essential oil, 68, 72, 78, 85, 127, 135, 158, 160, 168, 174, 181, 186, 190, 192, 193, 200, **254–255,** 312, 313

D

Douglas fir essential oil, 66, 67

E

East Indian geranium. *See* Palma rosa essential oil

Elecampane essential oil, 30

English chamomile. *See* Roman chamomile essential oil

Eucalyptus essential oil, 32, 67, 68, 81, 90, 92, 97, 99, 101, 102, 103, 104, 107, 108, 111, 115, 117, 135, 136, 159, 160, 165, 170, 183, 184, 194, 206, 222, **256–257,** 311, 312, 313

European mandarin. *See* Tangerine essential oil

Evening primrose carrier oil, 28, 67, 149, 159

Evening primrose essential oil, 61, 108

Everlasting oil. *See* Helichrysum essential oil

Eye bright. *See* Clary sage essential oil

F

False cinnamon. *See* Cassia essential oil

Fennel essential oil, 32, 33, 85, 142, 168, 192, 193, **257–258**

Fig leaf absolute essential oil, 30

Fir needle essential oil, 168

Frankincense essential oil, 56, 60, 68, 79, 81, 87, 99, 109, 110, 114, 115, 119, 120, 122, 126, 130, 136, 158, 168, 171, 186, 217, **259–260,** 311, 312, 313

G

Galbanum essential oil, 61

Geranium essential oil, 34, 67, 68, 69, 79, 93, 94, 109, 110, 117, 122, 141, 143, 145, 148, 149, 158, 164, 168, 192, 193, 204, 209, 212, 217, **260–262,** 311, 312, 313

German chamomile essential oil, 68, 75, 108, 117, 136, 165, 189, 192, **245–246,** 311, 312

Ginger essential oil, 12, 35, 36, 99, 110, 136, 143, 145, 146, 147, 152, 153, 154, 168, 217, **262–263,** 311, 312

Grapefruit essential oil, 35, 49, 85, 145, 146, 168, 192, 193, 207, 222, 223, **263–265**

Grape seed carrier oil, 15, 28–29, 93, 166, 211

Gum benzoin. *See* Benzoin essential oil

Gum thus. *See* Frankincense essential oil

H

Hazelnut carrier oil, 29

Helichrysum essential oil, 65, 76, 79, 80, 86, 89, 109, 110, 113, 126, 158, 166, 173, 179, 180, 181, 186, 189, **265,** 311, 312, 313

Ho leaf essential oil, 32

Hops essential oil, 34

Horseradish essential oil, 30

Hungarian chamomile. *See* German chamomile essential oil

Hyacinth essential oil, 34

Hyssop essential oil, 33, 74, 184, **267**

I

Immortelle. *See* Helichry-
   sum essential oil
Indian melissa oil.
   See Lemongrass
   essential oil
Indian verbena oil.
   See Lemongrass
   essential oil

J

Jaborandi essential oil, 30
Jamaica pepper. *See* Allspice essential oil
Jasmine essential oil, 36,
   142, 148, 168, 178, 200,
   202, **268–269**, 311,
   312, 313
Jojoba carrier oil, 29, 59,
   95, 104, 106, 110, 111,
   123, 134, 154, 162, 166,
   167, 169, 171, 187, 205,
   206, 207, 211, 225
Juniper berry essential
   oil, 36, 58, 85, 138, 159,
   192, 193, **269–270,**
   311, 312

K

Kayaputi. *See* Cajeput
   essential oil

L

Laurel. *See* Bay
   essential oil
Laurel essential oil, 32
Lavandin essential oil,
   270–271
Lavender essential oil, 34,
   58, 60, 61, 64, 66, 68,
   69, 72, 74, 75, 78, 80,
   81, 83, 86, 87, 88, 89,
   92, 93, 94, 97, 99, 100,
   101, 103, 106, 107, 108,
   111, 114, 115, 117, 119,
   120, 122, 123, 124, 126,
   129, 131, 132, 133, 136,
   139, 140, 141, 147, 149,

152, 155, 157, 158, 160,
   161, 165, 166, 168, 171,
   172, 173, 175, 176, 178,
   179, 180, 184, 185, 186,
   187, 192, 194, 200, 205,
   209, 210, 211, 217, 222,
   224, 226, **271–272,**
   311, 312, 313
   avoiding topical use of,
   for prepubesent
   boys, 16
Lemon balm. *See* Melissa
   essential oil
Lemon essential oil, 10,
   35, 49, 65, 78, 81, 82,
   85, 90, 92, 100, 103,
   115, 124, 145, 146, 157,
   158, 168, 171, 190, 205,
   209, 217, 222, 225,
   226, 229, **272–273,**
   311, 312, 313
Lemongrass essential
   oil, 32, 49, 65, 89, 158,
   167, 181, 183, 185, 222,
   225, **274**
Lemon verbena essential
   oil, 35, **276**
Lime essential oil, 35,
   49, 110, 111, 168, 209,
   276–277
Linden blossom essential
   oil, 34
Luban jawi. *See* Benzoin
   essential oil

M

Macadamia carrier oil, 29
Mace essential oil, 34
Madagarscar cinnamon.
   See Cinnamon essen-
   tial oil
Mandarin. *See* Tangerine
   essential oil
Mandarin essential oil,
   35, 49, 149, 168
Marigold oil. *See* Tagetes
   essential oil
Marjoram essential oil,
   34, 69, 72, 80, 84, 95,
   133, 134, 138, 143,
   145, 152, 162, 164,
   278–279

Massoia bark essential
   oil, 30
Meadow cumin. *See* Cara-
   way essential oil
Mediterranean bay. *See*
   Bay essential oil
Melasol. *See* Tea tree
   essential oil
Melilotus essential oil, 30
Melissa essential oil, 88,
   115, **279–280**
Melrose blend essential
   oil, 88
Motia. *See* Palma rosa
   essential oil
Muscatel sage. *See* Clary
   sage essential oil
Mustard essential oil, 30
Myrrh essential oil, 11, 60,
   61, 87, 89, 119, 136, 168,
   180, 210, **280–281**

N

Neroli essential oil, 34,
   61, 97, 114, 135, 142,
   149, 167, 168, 175, 176,
   281–283
Niaouli essential oil,
   283–284
Nutmeg essential oil, 32,
   34, 61, 120, 154, 168,
   218, **284–285**

O

Ocotea essential oil, 30
Oculus Christi. *See* Clary
   sage essential oil
Olibanum. *See* Frankin-
   cense essential oil
Olive carrier oil, 29, 31,
   62, 65, 72, 78, 82, 131,
   136, 181, 184, 189, 190,
   206, 207
Orange blossom oil. *See*
   Neroli essential oil
Orange essential oil, 10,
   35, 49, 158, 209, 217,
   285–286, 311, 312
Orange seed essential
   oil, 59

Oregano essential oil, 49, 59, 99, 115, 131, 170, 171, 185, 222

Ormenis flower essential oil, 34

P

Palma rosa essential oil, 108, 142, 168, **286–287**

Patchouli essential oil, 84, 89, 97, 154, 158, 165, 168, 200, 209, **287–288,** 311, 312, 313

Peppermint essential oil, 32, 36, 43, 62, 65, 67, 68, 69, 74, 78, 88, 90, 95, 97, 100, 101, 102, 108, 111, 113, 114, 115, 117, 123, 124, 125, 126, 127, 130, 134, 135, 136, 141, 145, 146, 150, 155, 158, 161, 168, 170, 171, 174, 183, 194, 206, 207, 210, 222, **288–289,** 311, 312

Petitgrain essential oil, 34, 168, **289–290**

Pimenta. *See* Allspice essential oil

Pimento oil. *See* Allspice essential oil

Pine essential oil, 103, 159, 160, 168, 174, 222, **290–292**

Primrose carrier oil, 67

Pure aloe vera gel, 84

R

Raven essential oil, 81

Ravensara blend, 88

Ravensara essential oil, 115

Red raspberry seed carrier oil, 180

Roman chamomile essential oil, 76, 80, 81, 88, 93, 97, 108, 133, 135, 141, 142, 149, 152, 158, 161, 165, 166, 168, 172, 175, 180, 184, **246–248,** 311, 312

Rose essential oil, 36, 61, 76, 161, 166, 168, 178, 189, 204, **292–293**

Rose geranium essential oil, **293–294**

Rose hip essential oil, 87

Rose hip seed essential oil, 64

Rosemary essential oil, 33, 36, 62, 72, 80, 84, 85, 92, 95, 97, 100, 115, 123, 134, 152, 158, 159, 185, 186, 187, 205, 222, **294–295,** 311, 312, 313

Rose otto essential oil, 66, 209

Rosewood essential oil, 108, 168, **296**

Rosha. *See* Palma rosa essential oil

Rue essential oil, 30

S

Safety
of essential oils, 32–34, 261
for babies, 34, 36
for children, 16, 34, 36, 139
for pets, 36
in pregnancy, 16, 34, 36, 231

Sage essential oil, 33, 72, 85, 104, 115, 117, 159, **297–299**

St. John's herb. *See* Helichrysum essential oil

Sandalwood essential oil, 34, 61, 66, 99, 108, 120, 158, 165, 168, 175, 176, 200, 225, **299–300**

Santolina essential oil, 30

Sassafras essential oil, 30, 32

Savin essential oil, 30

Scotch pine essential oil, 168

See bright. *See* Clary sage essential oil

Sesame seed carrier oil, 31

Seychelles cinnamon. *See* Cinnamon essential oil

Single chamomile. *See* German chamomile essential oil

Southernwood essential oil, 30

Spearmint essential oil, 168, 206, **300**

Spike lavender essential oil, 33, 113

Spikenard essential oil, 34, **301**

Spruce essential oil, 81, 168, 174

Star anise essential oil, 32, 168

Styrax essential oil, 30

Sunflower carrier oil, 78, 93, 190, 192

Sweet almond carrier oil, 31, 61, 78, 108, 117, 145, 169, 171, 175, 176, 180, 181, 190, 194, 203, 204, 210

Sweet bay. *See* Bay essential oil

Sweet cumin. *See* Aniseed essential oil

Sweet fennel essential oil, 36

Sweet marjoram essential oil, 36

Sweet orange essential oil, 114, 146, 168, 169

T

Tagetes essential oil, 35, 98, **301–302**

Tangerine essential oil, 10, 35, 49, 168, 178, 209, **302–303**

Tansy essential oil, 30

Tarragon essential oil, 127

Tasmanian blue gum. *See* Eucalyptus essential oil

Tea tree essential oil, 16, 34, 56, 68, 69, 71, 75, 78, 82, 84, 86, 88, 92, 93, 99, 103, 104, 107, 115, 116, 131, 132, 136, 139, 140, 158, 162, 165, 167, 170, 171, 184, 185, 187, 205, 207, 222, 223, 225, 226, **304–306,** 311, 312, 313

Thyme essential oil, 33, 49, 58, 90, 92, 99, 102, 104, 109, 110, 115, 123, 222, **306–307,** 311, 312, 313

Ti-trol. *See* Tea tree essential oil

Tonka bean essential oil, 30

True mandarin. *See* Tangerine essential oil

Turkish geranium. *See* Palma rosa essential oil

V
...

Valerian essential oil, 34

Vanilla essential oil, 148, 168, 200, 203, 206, 207, 217

Vegetable carrier oil, 68, 69, 81

Verbena essential oil, 30, 32

Vetiver essential oil, 34, 168, 169, **307**

Violet leaf essential oil, 61

W
...

Walnut carrier oil, 31

Weeping paperback. *See* Cajeput essential oil

Weeping tea tree. *See* Cajeput essential oil

Wheat germ carrier oil, 31–32, 176

White wood. *See* Cajeput essential oil

Wild orange essential oil, 211

Wintergreen essential oil, 67, 74, 81, 136, 154, 161, 174

Wormseed essential oil, 30

Wormwood essential oil, 30

Y
...

Yarrow essential oil, 106

Ylang-ylang essential oil, 34, 66, 129, 130, 133, 141, 158, 167, 168, 175, 176, 189, 200, **308–309,** 311, 312

Yuzu essential oil, 35

Oils of Aloha
Kukui oil (natural expeller pressed oil)

Dry skin
BURNS
ECZEMA
PSORIASIS
RADIATION BURNS

REMEDIES AND RECIPES INDEX

*__Boldface__ indicates a major discussion.

A
. . .

Abdominal pain, 246
Aches, **152–153,** 231, 257, 290, 307. *See also* Pain, muscle
Acid reflux, **56**
Acne, **56–59,** 232, 234, 239, 241, 251, 264, 274, 277, 286, 287, 290
Age spots, **59–61**
Aging skin, **61–64,** 286, 287, 296, 299, 301, 303
Agitation, 246, 254, 259, 271
Air freshener, **222**
Allergies, **64–65,** 232, 245
All-purpose cleaners, **222–223**
Anemia, **65–66**
Anger, 290, 292, 307
Animal bites, 306
Anorexia, 236, 238, 258, 284, 286
Anxiety, **66–67,** 236, 244, 245, 259, 267, 271, 278, 279, 281, 287, 308
Arthritis, **67–68,** 231, 232, 233, 234, 238, 239, 242, 243, 244, 248, 251, 253, 259, 265, 269, 272, 277, 278, 290, 295, 306, 307
Asthma, **68–69,** 232, 239, 241, 246, 251, 254, 259, 292
Astringents, **200**
Athlete's foot, **69–71,** 286

B
. . .

Back pain, **72–73**
Bath balls, **200–202**
Bathroom cleaner, **223**
Bath salts, **202–203**
Bathtub cleaner, **223–224**
Bee stings, **73–74**
Bites
    animal, 306
    insect, **132–133,** 232, 272, 277, 287, 290
    spider, **172**
    tick, **184–185**
Black toenail, **74–75**
Bleeding, 254
Blisters, **75–76**
Blood vessels, broken, **76–78**
Body butter, **203**
Body odor, **78**
Boils, **79**
Breast engorgement, 260
Bronchial congestion, 244, 299
Bronchitis, 231, 232, 234, 239, 241, 242, 254
Bruises, **79–80,** 241, 251
Bunions, **81–82**
Burns, **83,** 251, 271, 293

C
. . .

Calluses, **82, 84**
Cancer, **84**
Candles, **216**
Cardiac issues, 292
Catarrh, 231, 262
Cellulite, **85,** 258, 264, 269, 272, 277
Chafing, **85–86**

Chapped lips, **87**
Chicken pox, **88–89,** 256
Chicken skin, **89–90**
Chilblains, 234
Chills, 262
Circulatory issues, 233, 234, 238, 256, 260, 265, 272, 277, 284, 295
Cleaners
    all-purpose, **222–223**
    bathroom, **223**
    bathtub, **223–224**
    floor, **225**
    toilet, **226**
    window, **227**
Colds, **90–92,** 233, 234, 238, 239, 243, 248, 249, 253, 262, 264, 267, 270, 283, 296
Cold sores, **93–94,** 279
Colic, **94–95,** 231, 239, 241, 243, 267
Colitis, **95–97**
Conjunctivits, 292
Constipation, **97–98,** 232, 238, 272, 284
Corns, **98–99**
Coughs, **99,** 234, 241, 254, 270, 292, 296
    whooping, **193–194,** 231, 254
Cracked heels, **100–101**
Cramps, 230, 231, 253
    menstrual, **143–145**
Crohn's disease, **95–97**
Croup, **101–102**
Cuticle treatment, **204**
Cuts, **102–103,** 236, 251, 277, 290
Cystitis, **188,** 236
Cysts, ganglion, **120**

D

Dandruff, **103–104,** 304
Deodorant, **204**
Depression, 230, 234, 236,
   250, 264, 268, 276,
   279, 281, 287, 288, 292,
   293, 297, 299
Dermatitis, 297
Diabetes, **106**
Diaper rash, **106–107**
Diarrhea, **107,** 233, 243
Digestive issues, 239, 243,
   248, 250, 251, 255,
   258, 262, 265, 269,
   274, 276, 279, 280, 281,
   283, 284, 285, 286,
   288, 297, 300, 303
Diminished libido, **169,**
   278, 287, 296, 308
Dryer balls, **224**
Dry skin, **107–109,** 308
Dysplasia, 258

E

Eczema, **109–110,** 234,
   236, 245
Edema, 242
Emphysema, 254
Erectile dysfunction, 268
Excessive perspiration,
   160–161, 254, 290
Exhaustion, 238, 274, 286,
   290, 307

F

Fabric softener, **224**
Facial cleanser, **205**
Fainting, 284
Fatigue, **110,** 267, 290,
   300
Fever, **111–113,** 238, 239,
   243, 256, 262, 272,
   274, 277, 279, 286, 296
Fibromyalgia, **113–114**
Flatulence, **114,** 230, 231,
   241, 243, 253, 267
Floor cleaner, **225**

Flu, **115,** 233, 238, 242,
   243, 248, 249, 253,
   254, 264, 267, 270, 283
Fluid retention, 254, 267,
   269, 285, 287
Foot odor, **116–117**
Foot pain, **117–118**
Freckles, **118–120**
Furniture polish, **225**

G

Gall bladder issues,
   245, 246
Gallstones, 284
Ganglion cysts, **120**
Genitourinary issues, 267
Gout, **122,** 232, 242, 269,
   290, 295, 306
Grief, 292, 297

H

Hair, thinning, 233
Hair conditioner,
   205–206
Hair loss, **122–123,**
   233, 264
Hangover, **123–124,**
   231, 276
Hay fever, 246, 292. *See
   also* Allergies
Headaches, **124–125,** 255,
   257, 274, 281, 296
   migraine, **146–148,**
      231, 232, 253, 257,
      278, 279, 288, 295,
      300, 301
Head lice, **139–140,**
   260, 293
Heartburn, **56**
Heart palpitations,
   276, 281
Heels, cracked, **100–101**
Hemorrhoids, **126,**
   254, 280
Herpes, 272, 277
Hiccups, **126–127,** 258
High blood pressure, 272,
   279, 292, 308
Hives, **127–128**
Hormonal imbalance, 294

Hot flashes. *See* Meno-
   pause symptoms
Hyperactivity, 278
Hypertension, **129–130**

I

Immunosuppression,
   264, 285, 296
Indigestion, **130,** 230,
   231, 238, 267
Infections, 236, 239, 274,
   287, 304
   respiratory, 248
Inflammation, 245,
   256, 299
   joint, **136–138**
   skin, 259, 288
   testicle, **183–184**
Ingrown toenail, **131–132**
Insect bites, **132–133,**
   232, 272, 277, 287, 290
Insomnia, **133,** 250, 278,
   281, 285, 290, 301, 307
Intestinal issues, 295
Irritable bowel syndrome,
   134–135
Itch, jock, **135–136**
Itching, 241, 244, 246,
   299, 300

J

Jet lag, 274
Jock itch, **135–136**
Joint inflammation,
   136–138

K

Kidney issues, 250, 269

L

Labor-related issues, 250,
   268, 280
Lactation issues, 241, 255
Laryngitis, 239
Laundry detergent, **226**
Leg cramps, **138**
Lice, **139–140**
Lip balm, **206–207**

Lip gloss, **207**
Lips, chapped, **87**
Liver issues, 242, 245,
    258, 276, 292
Liver spots, **59–61**
Lyme disease, **184–185**

M
...

Malaria, 257
Mask, **209**
Measles, 257
Menopause symptoms,
    140–143, 245,
    250, 297
Menstrual cramps,
    143–145
Menstrual issues, 232,
    241, 245, 248, 250,
    259, 267, 269, 278,
    280, 288, 292, 297
Mental fatigue, 241, 253,
    288, 295
Metabolism, slow,
    145–146
Migraine, **146–148,** 231,
    232, 253, 257, 278,
    279, 288, 295, 300, 301
Moisturizer, **209–210**
Moodiness, **148–150**
Motion sickness, **150,** 262
    alleviating, **151**
Muscle aches, **152–153,**
    231, 257, 290, 307
Muscle fatigue, 264
Muscle pain, 231, 233,
    234, 238, 239, 250,
    270, 274, 278, 284,
    288, 295
Muscle spasms, 253
Muscle stiffness, 286

N
...

Nail growth oil, **210**
Nausea, **153–155,** 230,
    232, 243, 262, 271,
    288, 292
Neck stiffness, **155–157**
Nervous disorders, 232
Nervousness, 241

Neuralgia, 230, 233, 260,
    283, 288
Nosebleed, **157–158**

O
...

Obesity, 258, 264
Oily skin, **158,** 290, 294
Orchitis, **183–184**
Osteoporosis, **159–160**

P
...

Pain, 245, 251, 271. *See
    also* Aches
    abdominal, 246
    back, **72–73**
    foot, **117–118**
    muscle, 231, 233, 234,
        238, 239, 250, 270,
        274, 278, 284,
        288, 295
Perspiration, excess,
    160–161, 254, 290
Pillow spray, **217**
Poison ivy, **161–162**
Potpourri, **217–218**
Premenstrual syndrome,
    162–164, 246, 260
Prostate issues, 269
Prostatitis, 164–165
Psoriasis, **165–166,** 234,
    236, 239, 245, 246
Pulmonary
    congestion, 280

R
...

Rash, 234
    diaper, **106–107**
    skin, 246
Reproductive issues, 284,
    293, 297
Respiratory illnesses, 268,
    288, 302
Respiratory infections,
    248, 274, 283
Respiratory issues, 265,
    267, 271, 278, 290,
    295, 300, 304, 306

Restless leg syndrome,
    166–167
Rheumatoid arthritis, 257
Ringworm, **167,** 260

S
...

Sachets, **218**
Scalp issues, 241, 308
Scars, 265, 268, 281
Scar tissue, 234
Scented stationery, **219**
Sciatica, 306
Scrapes, **102–103,** 251,
    277, 290
Scrub, **211**
Sexual dysfunction,
    169, 276
Shampoo, **211–212**
Sinusitis, 239, 262, 280
Sinus pressure, **169–170**
Skin
    aging, **61–64,** 286, 287,
        296, 299, 301, 303
    blemishes, 271
    cancer, 179
    chicken, **89–90**
    dry, **107–109,** 308
    infections, 233
    inflammation, 259, 288
    irritation, 288
    issues, 258, 260, 268,
        269, 280, 300
    lesions, 265
    oily, **158,** 290, 294
    patch test, 15–16, 40
    puffiness and
        swelling, 295
    rashes, 262
    sensitivity of, 33
        testing for, 15–16
    sores, 262
    tags, **170–171**
    ulcers, 297
Sore throat, **171–172,**
    260, 262
Spider bites, **172**
Spider veins, **76**
Spleen issues, 258
Splinters, **173**
Sprains, **173–174**

Stationery, scented, **219**
Stiff neck, 297
Stings, bee, **73–74**
Stomach issues, 241
Stress, **174–176,** 230, 231,
     234, 236, 244, 250,
     253, 255, 259, 260,
     264, 269, 274, 276,
     278, 281, 285, 286,
     288, 290, 293, 299,
     300, 301, 307, 308
Stretch marks, **176–178,**
     268, 281
Sunburn, **178–181,**
     288, 304

T
. . .

Tendinitis, **181–183**
Tension, **174–176,** 230,
     231, 234, 236, 244,
     250, 253, 255, 269,
     285, 293, 299, 301, 308
Testicle inflammation,
     183–184

Tick bites, **184–185**
Tinnitus, **186–187**
Toenails
     black, **74–75**
     fungus on, **187–188**
     ingrown, **131–132**
Toilet cleaner, **226**
Toner, skin, **212**
Tonsillitis, 260

U
. . .

Ulcers, 260
     skin, 297
Urinary issues, 269
Urinary stones, 245
Urinary tract infections,
     188, 236, 239, 241,
     244, 259, 283
Urinary tract issues,
     290, 299
Urine retention, 264,
     294, 300

V
. . .

Varicose veins, **189–190,**
     254, 295
Vertigo, 231, 281, 288
Vomiting, 232, 239, 271

W
. . .

Warts, **190**
Wasp stings, **192**
Water retention, **192–193**
Whopping cough,
     193–194, 231, 254
Window cleaner, **227**
Wounds, 234, 236, 246,
     255, 259, 287, 294,
     297, 302, 304

INDEX

***Boldface** indicates a major discussion.

A

Abdominal pain, 246
Absolutes, 12
Aches, **152–153,** 231, 257, 290, 307. *See also* Pain, muscle
Acid reflux, **56**
Acne, **56–59,** 232, 234, 239, 241, 251, 264, 274, 277, 286, 287, 290
Acupressure, 45
  essential oils for, 45–46
Acupuncture, 45
  essential oils for, 45–46
Adulterated oil, 20
Age spots, **59–61**
Aging skin, **61–64,** 286, 287, 296, 299, 301, 303
Agitation, 246, 254, 259, 271
Air freshener, **222**
Ajowan essential oil, 30
Allergies, 232, 245
  seasonal, **64–65**
All-purpose cleaner, **222–223**
Allspice essential oil, 168, **230**
Almond oil, 15
Aloe vera carrier oil, 28, 179
Ambrette seed essential oil, 168
Amlodipine, 32
Amygdala, 14
Amyris essential oil, 168
Analgesics, 311
Anemia, **65–66**
Angelica essential oil, 35, 36, 162, 164
Anger, 290, 292, 307

Animal bites, 306
Anise. *See* Aniseed essential oil
Aniseed essential oil, 33, **230–231**
Anorexia, 236, 238, 258, 284, 286
Antidepressants, 311
Antifungal agents, 311
Anti-inflammatory agents, 311
Anti-scarring agents, 311
Antiseed essential oil, 32
Antiseptic agents, 312
Antispasmodic agents, 312
Antiviral aromatic herbs, 2
Anxiety, **66–67,** 236, 244, 245, 259, 267, 271, 278, 279, 281, 287, 293, 308
Aphrodisiac agents, 312
Aphrodisiac blends, essential oils for, 168
Apricot kernel carrier oil, 28, 62, 108, 130, 204
Aromatherapy, defined, 13
Aromatherapy-grade, 21
Aromatic methods, 39–45
Arthritis, **67–68,** 231, 232, 233, 234, 238, 239, 242, 243, 244, 248, 251, 253, 259, 265, 269, 272, 277, 278, 290, 295, 306, 307
Asarone, 32
Asthma, **68–69,** 232, 239, 241, 246, 251, 254, 259, 292
Astringents, **200,** 312
Athlete's foot, **69–71,** 286
Atomizers, 24
Aura Cacia products, 314
Avicenna, 11
Avocado carrier oil, 28, 61, 72, 108, 110, 120, 183

Ayurvedic medical practices, 1
Azob. *See* Hyssop essential oil

B

Babies, safety of essential oils for, 34, 36
Back pain, **72–73**
Balsam fir essential oil, 81, 168
Balsam of Peru essential oil, 30
Basil essential oil, 32, 33, 72, 95, 122, 134, 136, 138, 153, 155, 186, 192, 194, **232–233,** 311, 312
Bastard lavender. *See* Lavandin essential oil
Bath balls, **200–202**
Bathing, essential oils for, 49
Bathroom cleaner, **223**
Bath salts, **202–203**
Bathtub cleaners, **223–224**
Bay essential oil, 32, 33, **233–234**
Bee balm. *See* Melissa essential oil
Bee stings, **73–74**
Benjamin. *See* Benzoin essential oil
Benzoin essential oil, 34, **234–236**
Bergamot essential oil, 10, 35, 49, 66, 129, 130, 141, 146, 153, 154, 158, 168, 171, 188, 189, 209, 217, **236–238,** 311, 312, 313
Bible, 11

Bites
  animal, 306
  insect, **132–133,** 232,
    272, 277, 287, 290
  spider, **172**
  tick, **184–185**
Bitter almond essential
  oil, 30
Bitter orange essential oil,
  35, 49, 84
Black pepper essential
  oil, 84, 97, 153, 168,
  238–239, 311,
  312, 313
Black toenail, **74–75**
Bleeding, 254
Blenders, 25
Blisters, **75–76**
Blood vessels, broken,
  76–78
Blue chamomile. *See*
  German chamomile
  essential oil
Blue cypress essential oil,
  61, 120
Blue gum. *See* Eucalyptus
  essential oil
Body butter, **203**
Body odor, **78**
Boils, **79**
Bois de rose essential
  oil, 61
Boldo leaf essential oil, 30
Borage seed essential oil,
  61, 178
Bottles, 23
  clear glass, 22
  dusty, 22
Brands, essential oils,
  314–316
Breast engorgement, 260
Bronchial congestion,
  244, 299
Bronchitis, 231, 232, 234,
  239, 241, 242, 254
Bruises, **79–80,** 241, 251
Bubonic plague, 2
Buchu essential oil, 33
Bulking, 22–23
Bunions, **81–82**
Burns, **83,** 251, 271, 293

C
...

Cade oil crude essential
  oil, 30
Cajeput essential oil,
  239–241
Cajuput. *See* Cajeput
  essential oil
Calamus essential oil, 32
Calcium channel
  blocker, 32
Calendula carrier oil,
  28, 192
Calendula essential oil,
  80, 98
Calluses, **82, 84**
Camphor essential oil, 30,
  32, 33
Cancer, 32, **84**
  skin, 179
Candles, **216**
Caps
  loose, 22
  replacing tightly, 25–26
Caraway essential oil,
  241–242
Cardamom essential oil,
  97, 168
Cardiac issues, 292
Cardiac problems, 32–33
Carminative agents, 312
Carnation essential oil, 34
Carrier oils, 15, 47
  adding essential oils
    to, 15
  commonly available,
    26–29
Carrot carrier oil, 178
Carrot essential oil, 59,
  61, 104
Carrot seed carrier oil, 180
Carrot seed essential oil,
  64, 98, 108, 141, **242**
Cases, 23
Cassia bark. *See* Cassia
  essential oil
Cassia essential oil,
  33, **243**
Castor carrior oil, 119
Catarrh, 231, 262
Catnip essential oil, 133
Cayenne essential oil, 147

Cedarwood essential
  oil, 123, 141, 148, 168,
  194, 202, **244–245,**
  312, 313
Cellulite, **85,** 258, 264,
  269, 272, 277
Cepalic agents, 312
Ceylon cinnamon.
  See Cinnamon
  essential oil
Chafing, **85–86**
Chain of supply, 20
Chamomile essential oil,
  34, 36, 59, 66, 73, 74,
  75, 99, 109, 127, 142,
  153, 154, 164, 176,
  192, 202, 212, 217.
  See also German
  chamomile essential
  oil; Roman chamo-
  mile essential oil
Chapped lips, **87**
Chicken pox, **88–89,** 256
Chicken skin, **89–90**
Chilblains, 234
Children, safety of essen-
  tial oils for, 16, 34, 36
Chills, 262
Chinese cinnamon. *See*
  Cassia essential oil
Chinese parsley. *See* Coriander essential oil
Chlorophyll, 10
Chocolate peppermint
  essential oil, 168
Choomana poolu.
  See Lemongrass
  essential oil
Cinnamon essential oil,
  32, 33, 36, 49, 102, 115,
  145, 146, 148, 153, 168,
  217, 222, **248–249,**
  312, 313
Circulatory issues, 233,
  234, 238, 256, 260,
  265, 272, 277, 284, 295
Citronella essential oil,
  32, 133, 185, **249**
Clary sage essential oil,
  36, 58, 66, 72, 133,
  141, 143, 145, 158, 160,
  162, 164, 202, 209,
  250–251, 311, 312

Clary wort. *See* Clary sage
    essential oil
Cleaners
    all-purpose, **222–223**
    bathroom, **223**
    bathtub, **223–224**
    floor, **225**
    toilet, **226**
    window, **227**
Clear eye. *See* Clary sage
    essential oil
Clear glass bottles, 22
Clinical depression, 150
Clove essential oil, 32,
    33, 49, 67, 90, 92, 102,
    168, 169, 171, 173, 222,
    251–253
Coconut carrier oil, 59,
    60, 89, 90, 109, 113, 117,
    119, 142, 170, 171, 180,
    186, 202, 203, 204,
    206, 207, 211
Cold packs, 45
    benefits of, 46
    essential oils in, 46
Cold-pressing, 10
Colds, **90–92,** 233, 234,
    238, 239, 243, 248,
    249, 253, 262, 264,
    267, 270, 283, 296
Cold sores, **93–94,** 279
Colic, **94–95,** 231, 239,
    241, 243, 267
Colitis, **95–97**
Concrete, 10, 12
Conjunctivits, 292
Constipation, **97–98,**
    232, 238, 272, 284
Constituents, 26
Coriander essential oil,
    168, **253–254**
Corns, **98–99**
Costusroot essential
    oil, 30
Coughs, **99,** 234, 241, 254,
    270, 292, 296
    whooping, **193–194,**
    231, 254
Cracked heels, **100–101**
Cramps, 230, 231, 253
    menstrual, **143–145**
Crohn's disease, **95–97**
Croton essential oil, 30

Croup, **101–102**
Cumin essential oil, 35
Cuticle treatment, **204**
Cuts, **102–103,** 236, 251,
    277, 290
Cypress essential oil, 68,
    72, 78, 85, 127, 135,
    158, 160, 168, 174, 181,
    186, 190, 192, 193, 200,
    254–255, 312, 313
Cystatis, 188
Cystitis, **188,** 236
Cysts, ganglion, **120**

D
Dandruff, **103–104,** 304
Decongestants, 312
Deodorant, **204,** 312
Depression, 230, 234, 236,
    250, 264, 268, 276,
    279, 281, 287, 288, 292,
    293, 297, 299
    clinical, 150
Dermatitis, 297
Diabetes, **106**
Diaper rash, **106–107**
Diarrhea, **107,** 233, 243
Diffusers, 23–24, 34
    do-it-yourself, 44
    essential oils in a, 42
Digestive agents, 312
Digestive issues, 239, 243,
    248, 250, 251, 255,
    258, 262, 265, 269,
    274, 276, 279, 280, 281,
    283, 284, 285, 286,
    288, 297, 300, 303
Dill essential oil, 35
Diluents. *See* Dilutants
Dilutants, 20, 21
Diminished libido, **169,**
    278, 287, 296, 308
Direct inhalation, 39, 40
Discount oils, 13, 15
Disinfectants, 313
Distillation, 9–10
    hydrodiffusion, 9
    steam, 9
    water, 9
Diuretics, 313
dōTerra Aromatics, 40, 314

Douglas fir essential oil,
    66, 67
Driving, 34
Drop, size of, 43
Droppers, 24
Dryer balls, **224**
Dry skin, **107–109,** 308
Dusty bottles, 22
Dysplasia, 258

E
East Indian geranium.
    See Palma rosa
    essential oil
Eczema, **109–110,** 234,
    236, 245
Edema, 242
Einstein, Albert, 5
Elderly, caring for the, 33
Elecampane essential
    oil, 30
Emotion, essential oils
    and, 14
Emphysema, 254
English chamomile. *See*
    Roman chamomile
    essential oil
Epidermis, 85
Epilepsy, 33
Erectile dysfunction, 268
Esoteric Oils, 34, 314
Essential oils
    for acupuncture and
        acupressure, 45–46
    adding to carrier oils, 15
    adulterated, 20
    for aphrodisiac
        blends, 168
    avoiding, 30
    for bathing and
        showering, 49
    benefits of, 12–13
    burns and, 83
    in cold packs, 46
    concentration of, 15
    defined, 8
    in a diffuser, 42
    for direct and indirect
        inhalation, 39–40
    distillation of, 9–10
    effectiveness of, 55
    emotion and, 14

expression of, 10
in a facial steamer,
44–45
healing and, 11
in a humidifier, 40–41
for layering, 50
for massage, 45, 47
in a nebulizer, 43–44
safety of, 32–34, 261
for babies, 34, 36
for children, 16, 34,
36, 139
for pets, 36
in pregnancy, 16, 34,
36, 231
solvent extraction,
10, 12
storage of, in refrigerators, 26
tips for using, 13, 15–16
top 25, 311–313
understanding, 8
in a vaporizer, 41–42
in warm compresses, 46
Essential Vitality
products, 315
Ethanol, 12
Eucalyptus essential oil,
32, 67, 68, 81, 90, 92,
97, 99, 101, 102, 103,
104, 107, 108, 111, 115,
117, 135, 136, 159, 160,
165, 170, 183, 184, 194,
206, 222, **256–257,**
311, 312, 313
European mandarin.
See Tangerine
essential oil
Evening primrose carrier
oil, 28, 67, 149, 159
Evening primrose essential oil, 61, 108
Everlasting oil. *See* Helichrysum essential oil
Excessive perspiration,
160–161, 254, 290
Exhaustion, 238, 274, 286,
290, 307
Expectorants, 313
Expression, 10
Extenders, 20, 21
Extraction, 21

Extra-virgin olive oil, 29
Eye bright. *See* Clary sage
essential oil

F

Fabric softener, **224**
Facial cleansers, **205**
Facial steamer, essential
oils in a, 44–45
Fainting, 284
False cinnamon. *See* Cassia essential oil
Fatigue, **110,** 267, 290, 300
Fatty acids, 8
Febrifuge agents, 313
Fennel essential oil, 32,
33, 85, 142, 168, 192,
193, **257–258**
Fever, **111–113,** 238, 239,
243, 256, 262, 272,
274, 277, 279, 286, 296
Fibromyalgia, **113–114**
Fig leaf absolute essential
oil, 30
Fir needle essential oil, 168
First-degree burns, 83
Fixed oils, 8, 15–16
Flatulence, **114,** 230, 231,
241, 243, 253, 267
Floor cleaner, **225**
Flu, **115,** 233, 238, 242,
243, 248, 249, 253,
254, 264, 267, 270, 283
Fluid retention, 254, 267,
269, 285, 287
Folded oils, 23
Foot odor, **116–117**
Foot pain, **117–118**
Fragrance oil, 20
Frail persons, caring
for, 33
Frankincense, 11, 12
Frankincense essential
oil, 56, 60, 68, 79, 81,
87, 99, 109, 110, 114,
115, 119, 120, 122, 126,
130, 136, 158, 168, 171,
186, 217, **259–260,**
311, 312, 313
Freckles, **118–120**
Funnels, 24
Furniture polish, **225**

G

Galbanum essential oil, 61
Gall bladder issues,
245, 246
Gallstones, 284
Ganglion cysts, **120**
Genitourinary issues, 267
Geranium essential oil,
34, 67, 68, 69, 79, 93,
94, 109, 110, 117, 122,
141, 143, 145, 148, 149,
158, 164, 168, 192,
193, 204, 209, 212,
217, **260–262,** 311,
312, 313
German chamomile
essential oil, 68, 75,
108, 117, 136, 165, 189,
192, **245–246,** 311, 312
Ginger essential oil, 12,
35, 36, 99, 110, 136,
143, 145, 146, 147, 152,
153, 154, 168, 217,
262–263, 311, 312
Gout, **122,** 232, 242, 269,
290, 295, 306
Grapefruit essential oil,
35, 49, 85, 145, 146,
168, 192, 193, 207, 222,
223, **263–265**
Grape seed carrier oil, 15,
28–29, 93, 166, 211
Grief, 292, 297
Gum benzoin. *See* Benzoin essential oil
Gum thus. *See* Frankincense essential oil

H

Hair, thinning, 233
Hair conditioner,
205–206
Hair loss, **122–123,**
233, 264
Hangover, **123–124,**
231, 276
Hay fever, 246, 292. *See
also* Allergies
Hazelnut carrier oil, 29
Headache, **124–125,** 255,
257, 274, 281, 296

migraine, **146–148,** 231, 232, 253, 257, 278, 279, 288, 295, 300, 301

Head lice, **139–140,** 260, 293

Healing, essential oils and, 11

Heartburn, **56**

Heart palpitations, 276, 281

Heart problems, 32–33

Heels, cracked, **100–101**

Helichrysum essential oil, 65, 76, 79, 80, 86, 89, 109, 110, 113, 126, 158, 166, 173, 179, 180, 181, 186, 189, **265,** 311, 312, 313

Hemorrhoids, **126,** 254, 280

Hepatic problems, 33

Heritage Essential Oils products, 315

Herpes, 272, 277

Hexane, 12

Hiccups, **126–127,** 258

High blood pressure, 272, 279, 292, 308

Hives, **127–128**

Ho leaf essential oil, 32

Hops essential oil, 34

Hormonal imbalance, 294

Hormone influencers, 313

Horseradish essential oil, 30

Hot compresses, 45

Hot flashes. *See* Menopause symptoms

Humidifier, essential oils in a, 40–41

Hungarian chamomile. *See* German chamomile essential oil

Hyacinth essential oil, 34

Hydrocarbons, 8

Hydrodiffusion distillation, 9

Hyperactivity, 278

Hypercritical CO$_2$ extraction, 10, 12

Hypertension, **129–130**

Hyssop essential oil, 33, 74, 184, **267**

I

Immortelle. *See* Helichrysum essential oil

Immune system boosters, 313

Immunosuppression, 264, 285, 296

Indian melissa oil. *See* Lemongrass essential oil

Indian verbena oil. *See* Lemongrass essential oil

Indigestion, **130,** 230, 231, 238, 267

Indirect inhalation, 39, 40

Infections, 236, 239, 274, 287, 304
 respiratory, 248

Inflammation, 245, 256, 299
 joint, **136–138**
 skin, 259, 288
 testicle, **183–184**

Ingrown toenail, **131–132**

Inhalers, 25

Insect bites, **132–133,** 232, 272, 277, 287, 290

Insomnia, **133,** 250, 278, 281, 285, 290, 301, 307

Intestinal issues, 295

Irritable bowel syndrome, **134–135**

Itch, jock, **135–136**

Itching, 241, 244, 246, 299, 300

J

Jaborandi essential oil, 30

Jamaica pepper. *See* Allspice essential oil

Jasmine essential oil, 36, 142, 148, 168, 178, 200, 202, **268–269,** 311, 312, 313

Jet lag, 274

Jock itch, **135–136**

Joint inflammation, **136–138**

Jojoba carrier oil, 29, 59, 95, 104, 106, 110, 111, 123, 134, 154, 162, 166, 167, 169, 171, 187, 205, 206, 207, 211, 225

Juniper berry essential oil, 36, 58, 85, 138, 159, 192, 193, **269–270,** 311, 312

K

Kayaputi. *See* Cajeput essential oil

Keratosis pilaris, 89

Kidney issues, 250, 269

L

Labor-related issues, 250, 268, 280

Lactation issues, 241, 255

Laryngitis, 239

Laundry detergent, **226**

Laurel. *See* Bay essential oil

Laurel essential oil, 32

Lavandin essential oil, **270–271**

Lavender essential oil, 34, 58, 60, 61, 64, 66, 68, 69, 72, 74, 75, 78, 80, 81, 83, 86, 87, 88, 89, 92, 93, 94, 97, 99, 100, 101, 103, 106, 107, 108, 111, 114, 115, 117, 119, 120, 122, 123, 124, 126, 129, 131, 132, 133, 136, 139, 140, 141, 147, 149, 152, 155, 157, 158, 160, 161, 165, 166, 168, 171, 172, 173, 175, 176, 178, 179, 180, 184, 185, 186, 187, 192, 194, 200, 205, 209, 210, 211, 217, 222, 224, 226, **271–272,** 311, 312, 313
 avoiding topical use of, for prepubesent boys, 16

Layering, essential oils for, 50
Leg cramps, **138**
Lemon balm. *See* Melissa essential oil
Lemon essential oil, 10, 35, 49, 65, 78, 81, 82, 85, 90, 92, 100, 103, 115, 124, 145, 146, 157, 158, 168, 171, 190, 205, 209, 217, 222, 225, 226, 229, **272–273,** 311, 312, 313
Lemongrass essential oil, 32, 49, 65, 89, 158, 167, 181, 183, 185, 222, 225, **274**
Lemon verbena essential oil, 35, **276**
Lice, **139–140,** 260, 293
Limbic system, 14
Lime essential oil, 35, 49, 110, 111, 168, 209, **276–277**
Linden blossom essential oil, 34
Lip balm, **206–207**
Lip gloss, **207**
Lips, chapped, **87**
Liver issues, 242, 245, 258, 276, 292
Liver problems, 33
Liver spots, **59–61**
Loose caps, 22
Luban jawi. *See* Benzoin essential oil
Lyme disease, **184–185**

M
• • •

Macadamia carrier oil, 29
Mace essential oil, 34
Maceration, 26
Madagarscar cinnamon. *See* Cinnamon essential oil
Malaria, 257
Mandarin. *See* Tangerine essential oil
Mandarin essential oil, 35, 49, 149, 168
Marigold oil. *See* Tagetes essential oil

Marjoram essential oil, 34, 69, 72, 80, 84, 95, 133, 134, 138, 143, 145, 152, 162, 164, **278–279**
Masks, **209**
Massage, essential oils for, 45, 47
Massoia bark essential oil, 30
Meadow cumin. *See* Caraway essential oil
Measles, 257
Medicine well, 41
Mediterranean bay. *See* Bay essential oil
Melanoma, 179
Melasol. *See* Tea tree essential oil
Melilotus essential oil, 30
Melissa essential oil, 88, 115, **279–280**
Melrose blend essential oil, 88
Menopause symptoms, **140–143,** 245, 250, 297
Menstrual cramps, **143–145**
Menstrual issues, 232, 241, 245, 248, 250, 259, 267, 269, 278, 280, 288, 292, 297
Mental fatigue, 241, 253, 288, 295
Metabolism, **145–146**
Methane, 13
Methanol, 12
Methyl chavicol, 32
Methyll, 32
Migraine, **146–148,** 231, 232, 253, 257, 278, 279, 288, 295, 300, 301
Moisturizers, **209–210**
Moodiness, **148–150**
Motia. *See* Palma rosa essential oil
Motion sickness, **150,** 262
alleviating, **151**
Mountain Rose Herbs products, 315

Multi-level marketing (MLM) companies, 21–22
Muscatel sage. *See* Clary sage essential oil
Muscle aches, **152–153,** 231, 257, 290, 307
Muscle fatigue, 264
Muscle pain, 231, 233, 234, 238, 239, 250, 270, 274, 278, 284, 288, 295
Muscle spasms, 253
Muscle stiffness, 286
Mustard essential oil, 30
Myrrh essential oil, 11, 60, 61, 87, 89, 119, 136, 168, 180, 210, **280–281**

N
• • •

Nail growth oil, **210**
National Association for Holistic Aromatherapy, 13
Native American Nutritionals products, 315
Natural disasters, 1
Nature-identical oil, 20
Nausea, **153–155,** 230, 232, 243, 262, 271, 288, 292
Neat, 39
Nebulizer, 23–24, 34
essential oils in a, 43–44
Neck stiffness, **155–157**
Nelson, Nina, 211
Neroli essential oil, 34, 61, 97, 114, 135, 142, 149, 167, 168, 175, 176, **281–283**
Nervous disorders, 232
Nervousness, 241
Neuralgia, 230, 233, 260, 283, 288
Niaouli essential oil, **283–284**
North American Herb and Spice products, 316
Nosebleed, **157–158**

Nutmeg essential oil, 32, 34, 61, 120, 154, 168, 218, **284–285**

O
. . .

Obesity, 258, 264
Ocotea essential oil, 30
Oculus Christi. *See* Clary sage essential oil
Oily skin, **158**, 290, 294
Olfaction, 14
Olfactory bulb, 14
Olfactory epithelium, 14
Olfactory membrane, 14
Olibanum. *See* Frankincense essential oil
Olive carrier oil, 29, 31, 62, 65, 72, 78, 82, 131, 136, 181, 184, 189, 190, 206, 207
Orange blossom oil. *See* Neroli essential oil
Orange essential oil, 10, 35, 49, 158, 209, 217, **285–286**, 311, 312
Orange seed essential oil, 59
Orchitis, **183–184**
Oregano essential oil, 49, 59, 99, 115, 131, 170, 171, 185, 222
Ormenis flower essential oil, 34
Osteoporosis, **159–160**
Over-the-counter medications, 16

P
. . .

Pain, 245, 251, 271. *See also* Aches
abdominal, 246
back, **72–73**
foot, **117–118**
muscle, 231, 233, 234, 238, 239, 250, 270, 274, 278, 284, 288, 295
Palma rosa essential oil, 108, 142, 168, **286–287**

Parsley seed oil, 30
Patchouli essential oil, 84, 89, 97, 154, 158, 165, 168, 200, 209, **287–288,** 311, 312, 313
Peppermint essential oil, 32, 36, 43, 62, 65, 67, 68, 69, 74, 78, 88, 90, 95, 97, 100, 101, 102, 108, 111, 113, 114, 115, 117, 123, 124, 125, 126, 127, 130, 134, 135, 136, 141, 145, 146, 150, 155, 158, 161, 168, 170, 171, 174, 183, 194, 206, 207, 210, 222, **288–289,** 311, 312
Perfume oil, 21
Perfumes, 13
Perspiration, excess, **160–161,** 254, 290
Petitgrain essential oil, 34, 168, **289–290**
Petroleum ether, 12
Pets, safety of essential oils, 36
Photosensitizing oils, 33, 35
Phototoxicity, 33, 35
Pillow spray, **217**
Pimenta. *See* Allspice essential oil
Pimento oil. *See* Allspice essential oil
Pine essential oil, 103, 159, 160, 168, 174, 222, **290–292**
Pipettes, 24
Poison ivy, **161–162**
Potpourri, **217–218**
Pregnancy, safety of essential oils in, 16, 34, 36, 231
Premenstrual syndrome, **162–164,** 246, 260
Primrose carrier oil, 67
Prostate issues, 269
Prostatitis, **164–165**
Psoriasis, **165–166,** 234, 236, 239, 245, 246
Pulmonary congestion, 280

Pure essential oils, 20, 21
Pure aloe vera gel, 84
Pure olive oil, 31

R
. . .

Rash, 234
diaper, **106–107**
skin, 246
Raven essential oil, 81
Ravensara blend, 88
Ravensara essential oil, 115
Receptor neurons, 14
Reconstituted oils, 23
Rectified oils, 23
Redistilled oils, 23
Red raspberry seed carrier oil, 180
Refrigerator, storage of essential oils in, 26
Reproductive issues, 284, 293, 297
Respiratory illnesses, 268, 288, 302
Respiratory infections, 248, 274, 283
Respiratory issues, 265, 267, 271, 278, 290, 295, 300, 304, 306
Restless leg syndrome, **166–167**
Rheumatoid arthritis, 257
Ringworm, **167,** 260
Roman chamomile essential oil, 76, 80, 81, 88, 93, 97, 108, 133, 135, 141, 142, 149, 152, 158, 161, 165, 166, 168, 172, 175, 180, 184, **246–248,** 311, 312
Rose essential oil, 36, 61, 76, 161, 166, 168, 178, 189, 204, **292–293**
Rose geranium essential oil, **293–294**
Rose hip essential oil, 87
Rose hip seed essential oil, 64
Rosemary essential oil, 33, 36, 62, 72, 80, 84, 85, 92, 95, 97, 100, 115, 123, 134, 152, 158,

159, 185, 186, 187, 205,
222, **294–295,** 311,
312, 313
Rose otto essential oil,
66, 209
Rosewood essential oil,
108, 168, **296**
Rosha. *See* Palma rosa
essential oil
Rubefacients, 313
Rue essential oil, 30

S

Sachets, **218**
Safety of essential oils,
32–34, 261
for babies, 34, 36
for children, 16, 34,
36, 139
for pets, 36
in pregnancy, 16, 34,
36, 231
Safrole, 32
Sage essential oil, 33, 72,
85, 104, 115, 117, 159,
297–299
St. John's herb. *See* Heli-
chrysum essential oil
Sandalwood essential oil,
34, 61, 66, 99, 108, 120,
158, 165, 168, 175, 176,
200, 225, **299–300**
Santolina essential oil, 30
Sassafras essential oil,
30, 32
Savin essential oil, 30
Scalp issues, 241, 308
Scars, 234, 265, 268, 281
Scentastics 2
products, 316
Scented stationery, **219**
Sciatica, 306
Scotch pine essential
oil, 168
Scrapes, **102–103,** 251,
277, 290
Scrubs, **211**
Second-degree burns, 83
Sedatives, 313
See bright. *See* Clary sage
essential oil

Sensitivity, 33
testing skin for, 15–16
Sesame seed carrier oil, 31
Sexual dysfunction,
169, 276
Seychelles cinnamon.
See Cinnamon essen-
tial oil
Shalom Mama blog, 211
Shampoo, **211–212**
Shopping, 19–23
Showering, essential oils
for, 49
Single chamomile. *See*
German chamomile
essential oil
Sinusitis, 239, 262, 280
Sinus pressure, **169–170**
Skin
aging, **61–64,** 286, 287,
296, 299, 301, 303
blemishes, 271
cancer, 179
chicken, **89–90**
dry, **107–109,** 308
infections, 233
inflammation, 259, 288
irritation, 288
issues, 258, 260, 268,
269, 280, 300
lesions, 265
oily, **158,** 290, 294
patch test, 15–16, 40
puffiness and
swelling, 295
rashes, 262
sensitivity of, 33
testing for, 15–16
sores, 262
tags, **170–171**
ulcers, 297
Solvent extraction, 10, 12
Solvents, 12
Sore throat, **171–172,**
260, 262
Southernwood essential
oil, 30
Spearmint essential oil,
168, 206, **300**
Spider bites, **172**
Spider veins, **76**

Spike lavender essential
oil, 33, 113
Spikenard essential oil,
34, **301**
Spleen issues, 258
Splinters, **173**
Sprains, **173–174**
Spruce essential oil, 81,
168, 174
Star anise essential oil,
32, 168
Stationery, scented, **219**
Steam distillaton, 9–10
Stiff neck, 297
Stimulants, 313
Stings, bee, **73–74**
Stomach issues, 241
Storage, 25–26
Stress, **174–176,** 230, 231,
234, 236, 244, 250,
253, 255, 259, 260,
264, 269, 274, 276,
278, 281, 285, 286,
288, 290, 293, 299,
300, 301, 307, 308
Stretch marks, **176–178,**
268, 281
Styrax essential oil, 30
Sugar scrub, 49
Sunburn, **178–181,** 288, 304
Sunflower carrier oil, 78,
93, 190, 192
Sweet almond carrier
oil, 31, 61, 78, 108, 117,
145, 169, 171, 175, 176,
180, 181, 190, 194, 203,
204, 210
Sweet bay. *See* Bay essential oil
Sweet cumin. *See* Aniseed
essential oil
Sweet fennel essential
oil, 36
Sweet marjoram essential
oil, 36
Sweet orange essential
oil, 114, 146, 168, 169
Synthetic fragrance, 21
Syringes, 24

T
...

Tagetes essential oil, 35, 98, **301–302**

Tangerine essential oil, 10, 35, 49, 168, 178, 209, **302–303**

Tansy essential oil, 30

Tarragon essential oil, 127

Tasmanian blue gum. *See* Eucalyptus essential oil

Tea tree essential oil, 16, 34, 56, 68, 69, 71, 75, 78, 82, 84, 86, 88, 92, 93, 99, 103, 104, 107, 115, 116, 131, 132, 136, 139, 140, 158, 162, 165, 167, 170, 171, 184, 185, 187, 205, 207, 222, 223, 225, 226, **304–306**, 311, 312, 313
  avoiding topical use of, for prepubesent boys, 16

Tendinitis, **181–183**

Tension, **174–176**, 230, 231, 234, 236, 244, 250, 253, 255, 269, 285, 293, 299, 301, 308

Terpenes, 8, 10, 12

Testicle inflammation, **183–184**

Thalamus, 14

Therapeutic-grade essential oils, 2, 21

Third-degree burns, 83

Thyme essential oil, 33, 49, 58, 90, 92, 99, 102, 104, 109, 110, 115, 123, 222, **306–307**, 311, 312, 313

Tick bites, **184–185**

Tinnitus, **186–187**

Ti-trol. *See* Tea tree essential oil

Toenails
  black, **74–75**
  fungus on, **187–188**
  ingrown, **131–132**

Toilet cleaner, **226**

Toner, skin, **212**

Tonics, 313

Tonka bean essential oil, 30

Tonsillitis, 260

Tools and equipment, 23–26

Topical methods, 45–50

True mandarin. *See* Tangerine essential oil

Turkish geranium. *See* Palma rosa essential oil

U
...

Ulcers, 260
  skin, 297

Urinary issues, 269

Urinary stones, 245

Urinary tract infections, **188**, 236, 239, 241, 244, 259, 283

Urinary tract issues, 290, 299

Urine retention, 264, 294, 300

Urushiol, 161

V
...

Valerian essential oil, 34

Vanilla essential oil, 148, 168, 200, 203, 206, 207, 217

Vaporizer, essential oils in, 41–42

Varicose veins, **189–190**, 254, 295

Vegetable carrier oil, 68, 69, 81

Verbena essential oil, 30, 32

Vertigo, 231, 281, 288

Vetiver essential oil, 34, 168, 169, **307**

Vials, 23

Violet leaf essential oil, 61

Virgin olive oil, 29, 31

Vitamin E, 31–32

Volatile organic compounds (VOCs), 13, 14

Vomiting, 232, 239, 271

Vulnerary, 313

W
...

Walnut carrier oil, 31

Warm compresses
  essential oils in, 46
  making, 48

Warts, **190**

Wasp stings, **192**

Water-and-steam distillation, 9

Water distillation, 9

Water retention, **192–193**

Weeping paperback. *See* Cajeput essential oil

Weeping tea tree. *See* Cajeput essential oil

Western apothecary, 1

Wheat germ carrier oil, 31–32, 176

White wood. *See* Cajeput essential oil

Whopping cough, **193–194**, 231, 254

Wild orange essential oil, 211

Window cleaner, **227**

Wintergreen essential oil, 67, 74, 81, 136, 154, 161, 174

Wormseed essential oil, 30

Wormwood essential oil, 30

Wounds, 234, 236, 246, 255, 259, 287, 294, 297, 302, 304

Y
...

Yarrow essential oil, 106

Ylang-ylang essential oil, 34, 66, 129, 130, 133, 141, 158, 167, 168, 175, 176, 189, 200, **308–309**, 311, 312

Young Living products, 88, 316

Yuzu essential oil, 35

9 780989 558693